FINDING YOUR SEXUAL VOICE

Finding Your Sexual Voice promotes the genuine understanding of strong female sexuality and empowers women to value desire, pleasure, eroticism, and satisfaction. The book confronts myths and misunderstandings about female sexuality, especially desire, and encourages an increased understanding of healthy couple sexuality so that the woman and man can be intimate and erotic allies.

Each chapter includes a detailed psychosexual exercise, as well as a range of motivating case studies, to help women discover their sexual style and value their sexual voice. The guide also expands the concept of sex to include sensual, playful, and erotic touch, and emphasizes the multiple roles and meanings of the Good Enough Sex (GES) model.

This accessible and powerful book is pro-female, pro-couple, and pro-sexuality, and will be valuable reading for women, from 25–85, looking to build strong, resilient desire and to embrace female sexuality. It will also be of use to couples who are dealing with sexual dissatisfaction, as well as all mental health professionals involved in the fields of marriage, couple, and sex therapy.

Barry McCarthy is a Professor of Psychology at American University, a Diplomate in Clinical Psychology, a Diplomate in Sex Therapy, and a Certified Couple Therapist. He has published over 115 professional articles, 32 book chapters, and 17 books. He has presented over 450 professional workshops nationally and internationally. In 2016, he received the SSTAR Masters and Johnson award for lifetime contributions to the sex therapy field.

Emily J. McCarthy received a B.S. degree in speech communication, and her writing and wisdom provides a balanced, humanistic perspective. This is Emily and Barry's 13th co-authored book.

FINDING YOUR SEXUAL VOICE
Celebrating Female Sexuality

Barry McCarthy
Emily J. McCarthy

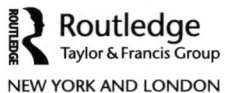

Routledge
Taylor & Francis Group
NEW YORK AND LONDON

First published 2019
by Routledge
52 Vanderbilt Avenue, New York, NY 10017

and by Routledge
2 Park Square, Milton Park, Abingdon, Oxon, OX14 4RN

Routledge is an imprint of the Taylor & Francis Group, an informa business

© 2019 Taylor & Francis

The right of Barry McCarthy and Emily J. McCarthy to be identified as authors of this work has been asserted by them in accordance with sections 77 and 78 of the Copyright, Designs and Patents Act 1988.

All rights reserved. No part of this book may be reprinted or reproduced or utilised in any form or by any electronic, mechanical, or other means, now known or hereafter invented, including photocopying and recording, or in any information storage or retrieval system, without permission in writing from the publishers.

Trademark notice: Product or corporate names may be trademarks or registered trademarks, and are used only for identification and explanation without intent to infringe.

Library of Congress Cataloging-in-Publication Data

Names: McCarthy, Barry W., 1943– author. | McCarthy, Emily J., author.
Title: Finding your sexual voice : celebrating female sexuality / Barry McCarthy, Emily J. McCarthy.
Description: New York, NY : Routledge, 2019. | Includes bibliographical references and index.
Identifiers: LCCN 2018035431 (print) | LCCN 2018037533 (ebook) | ISBN 9780429446078 (E-book) | ISBN 9781138333260 (hardback) | ISBN 9781138333277 (pbk.)
Subjects: LCSH: Sex instruction for women. | Couples—Sexual behavior. | Sex in marriage. | Sexual excitement.
Classification: LCC HQ46 (ebook) | LCC HQ46 .M37 2019 (print) | DDC 613.9/54—dc23
LC record available at https://lccn.loc.gov/2018035431

ISBN: 978-1-138-33326-0 (hbk)
ISBN: 978-1-138-33327-7 (pbk)
ISBN: 978-0-429-44607-8 (ebk)

Typeset in Perpetua
by Apex CoVantage, LLC

CONTENTS

1	The War Between Women and Men	1
2	The New Sexual Mantra: Desire/Pleasure/Eroticism/Satisfaction	15
3	First-Class Female Sexuality	31
4	Integrating Intimacy, Pleasuring, and Eroticism	45
5	Desire: The Core of Sexuality	59
6	Nondemand Pleasuring	73
7	Integrated Eroticism	87
8	Satisfaction: More than Orgasm	101
9	The Good Enough Sex (GES) Model	115
10	Developing Your Couple Sexual Style	131
11	Women and Men as Intimate and Erotic Allies	145
12	Satisfying, Secure, and Sexual Marriage	159

Appendix A: Choosing a Sex, Couple, or Individual Therapist   171
Appendix B: Suggested Readings   173
References   175

1

THE WAR BETWEEN WOMEN AND MEN

If you sit at a bar, especially after midnight, and listen to men talk about women and sex it is very discouraging. The theme is the inherent war between men and women, with sex as the battlefield. Men complain that women are "cock teasers" and use sex to manipulate. The message is that a "real man is willing and able to have sex with any woman, any time, any place." When she says no, she makes him a "loser," especially in the eyes of male peers. The sex game is about power, control, and manipulation. Sex, especially intercourse, is the man's domain. The woman has the role of sexual gatekeeper—the power of "no." If they have sex he's won, if not she's won.

The traditional male—female double standard has clear rules. However, the double standard is destructive for adult women and for the couple (Metz, Epstein, & McCarthy, 2017). Ultimately, it is destructive for the man since performance pressure subverts male sexual confidence and function. A little-known fact is that when couples stop being sexual, whether at 40, 60, or 80, it is almost always the man's choice made because he has lost confidence with erections, intercourse, and orgasm (McCarthy & Metz, 2008).

He cannot live up to the demands of the autonomous perfect sex performance model. The medical and drug company answer is to provide a medication, injection, or prosthesis to guarantee perfect sex performance. The message is not to turn to the woman and share pleasure, but to turn toward a bio-medical solution to guarantee individual sex performance.

Is autonomous, performance-oriented sex the right model for you as a woman? The double standard emphasizes sex as an all or nothing performance—he must always have an erection, intercourse, and orgasm. You should always have an orgasm (during intercourse). In contrast, the Good Enough Sex (GES) model emphasizes sexuality as a couple process of giving and receiving pleasure-oriented touching. GES is the healthy model for women, men, couples, and the culture (Metz & McCarthy, 2012).

Sexuality is intimate and interactive with a range of roles, meanings, and outcomes. Although arousal, intercourse, and orgasm are valued, this is not the core of healthy female and couple sexuality. Sexual experiences involving mutual, synchronous desire/pleasure/eroticism/satisfaction are most highly valued and rightly so. In addition, GES values the variability and flexibility of couple sexuality. Sexuality certainly involves intercourse but is more than intercourse. Sexuality involves sensual, playful, and erotic touch in addition to intercourse. Our theme is that intimate, interactive, pleasure-oriented couple sexuality is much superior to the male autonomous, individual sex performance model.

Ending the War

We strongly advocate confronting and changing the traditional dialogue about women, men, couples, and sexuality. Rather than sex being the battleground where one loses, we advocate a respectful, trusting, equitable relationship between the woman and man. Your relationship thrives when you view each other as intimate and erotic allies. We advocate for the female—male equity model for your emotional and sexual relationship. This is particularly valuable for adults in a married or partnered relationship.

Sexuality is as valuable for women as for men. The role of healthy sexuality is to energize the couple bond and reinforce feelings of desire and desirability. Rather than sexuality having a dramatic or disruptive role, it has a 15–20% positive role as a shared pleasure, a means to deepen and reinforce intimacy, and a tension reducer to deal with the stresses of a shared relationship and the vicissitudes of life (McCarthy & McCarthy, 2014).

The female—male equity model is very different than the double standard. Women and men are equitable life partners who respect and trust each other to share emotional and sexual intimacy. An equitable relationship involves sexual attitudes, behaviors, and emotions. Your partner respects you and accepts you as a unique person with strengths and vulnerabilities. The manipulation and game-playing which is so prevalent in double standard relationships is eliminated. What your partner says to you is congruent with what he says to male friends. Is this too idealistic? Equity functions best in a respectful, trusting, intimate relationship. It is challenging and difficult when discussing male—female issues in groups, especially same gender groups. In male groups, the peer pressure is to make jokes about women and sex or "one-up" each other. In female groups, the peer pressure is to complain about and demonize males. Neither dialogue promotes respect or understanding. The equity model encourages a serious, respectful dialogue, avoiding stereotypes and put-downs. Rather than giving the "socially desirable" response, it asks you and your partner to engage in a serious, respectful dialogue about gender and sexuality.

In adult sexual relationships there are many more similarities than differences between women and men (Hyde, 2005). This is true not just for intellectual and behavioral dimensions, but emotional and sexual similarities. The prime example is sharing the goal of a satisfying, secure, and sexual relationship.

In the traditional double standard, males valued sex and females valued intimacy. In the equity model both the woman and man value sexuality and intimacy. Of course, it is important to recognize psychological, biological, and relational differences. The challenge is to build a fully functioning relationship, including emotional and sexual equity. Males have lower expectations for an intimate relationship, with sex viewed as the reward for being married. The challenge for the man is to accept the woman as his partner, value intimacy and pleasuring, and reinforce a satisfying, secure bond. The challenge for the woman is to integrate your erotic voice into couple sexuality, confront the put-down approach to males and male sexuality, value your partner as an intimate and erotic ally, and replace the romantic love/passionate sex/idealization phase with a mature intimacy, integrated sexuality, and an equitable partnership (Sims & Meana, 2010).

The equity model asks a great deal of the woman, man, and couple. It is worth it because equity results in greater psychological, relational, and sexual growth and satisfaction. In addition, the equity model has scientific support which is not true of the double standard. Gender equity is a challenge to implement and requires thought, communication, and energy, but is rewarding for the woman, man, couple, and culture.

Wars are Hard to End

Culturally, the war between men and women has a long and painful history with personal, relational, and sexual horror stories that cost women dearly and caused great disruption. The history and grievances are a major factor in keeping the war between men and women going. A powerful example is the issue of rape. Rape has a long history and been used as a weapon of war (an example is the Yugoslavian conflict between Serbs, Croats, and Bosnians). An extreme position is the belief that all men are potential rapists. Can gender conflicts be resolved and the wounds healed?

A psychological adage is that you can learn from the past, but you cannot change the past. Life is better lived in the present with planning for the future rather than continuing to fight battles from the past. Refighting male—female sexual wars has little value. What has value is to establish a new model of female—male equity and within that reinforce desire/pleasure/eroticism/satisfaction. This meets the needs of the woman, man, and couple (Muise & Impett, 2015) and is a core theme throughout the book.

Melinda and Richard

Twenty-six-year-old Melinda and 24-year-old Richard were a volatile, demoralized couple of three years. They agreed to participate in a ten-session semi-structured, skill-based pre-marital program. Previously, they had attended group therapy and a short, unsatisfactory couple counseling.

Melinda graduated college as a woman's study major and worked as an organizational consultant while Richard was an IT professional. Their dynamic illustrated the typical male—female power struggle. Melinda accused Richard of being a "Neanderthal" who didn't understand himself or emotions and was sexually repressed. Richard described Melinda to male friends as a "touchy-feely addict and an emotional tiger." They were a sexually volatile couple. Richard teased Melinda that if she thought he was sexually inhibited, why she was so desirous and orgasmic. Melinda countered saying why couldn't he be a "new man" who shared intimacy and pleasuring—why did each experience have to end in intercourse? He felt sex was more fun when she was angry because it was so dramatic. Verbal conflict was foreplay for passionate sex. Melinda disliked this explanation, saying he thought like a repressed computer engineer, not a healthy man. Their attack—counterattack pattern continued unabated.

In entering the pre-marital program, they had very different agendas. Melinda wanted Richard to increase emotional and sexual awareness (i.e. realize she was right) so he would be the ideal life partner. Richard's agenda was confused and confusing. Ideally, he wanted a satisfying, secure, and sexual marriage, but was not at all sure he could achieve this. He feared Melinda was not the right woman for him with her social/political approach to gender, sex, and marriage. He especially worried about being the statistic he had seen in two of his friends—the woman leaves in less than two years because she was disappointed in the man and marriage. Based on his family model, Richard believed that the best aspect of the traditional male role was being the solid husband and father who provides marital, financial, and family stability.

The pre-marital program focused on attitudes, behaviors, and emotions which promote a satisfying, secure marriage. It stayed away from abstract/philosophical arguments, but did confront the male—female double standard and power struggles. The focus was on communication, problem-solving, and conflict-resolution skills. Marriage was presented as a respectful, trusting commitment based on a positive influence process. Being in a healthy marriage brings out the best in each person. You are a better person because you are married to this spouse. As with most marriage programs, the focus was on communication and emotional intimacy rather than sexuality.

Richard needed to be involved with relational issues, not just reactive to Melinda. He couldn't be governed by fears about women generally, and Melinda specifically. How much did he value a respectful, trusting relationship and was he open to a marital commitment? Richard wanted them to develop a genuine couple sexual style which integrates intimacy and eroticism rather than depending on sexual drama. Emotional intimacy nurtures the couple bond-awareness that the spouse cares about you and is responsive to your needs as well as "has your back." Sexual intimacy energizes the bond and reinforces feelings of desire and desirability. Melinda wanted a satisfying, secure, and sexual marriage.

The skill focus in the sessions and homework facilitated Melinda's and Richard's engagement in the change process. All individuals and couples have strengths and vulnerabilities. This was particularly motivating for Melinda—previously she'd seen only her strengths and Richard's vulnerabilities. Richard found the emphasis on skills training, including emotional vulnerability and empathic communication, of great value. To reach his goal of a secure family, a solid marriage was the foundation. He needed to increase respect and trust with Melinda if they were to be a healthy couple and create a cohesive family.

They'd fallen into the classic pursuer—distancer power struggle. Melinda did not just pursue Richard; she tried to coerce him to change. She did not believe that she could positively influence him and was afraid of being taken advantage of.

In creating an equitable emotional and sexual relationship, you have to confront the traditional double standard and break the gender power struggle. In healthy adult relationships there is recognition that intellectually, behaviorally, emotionally, and sexually there are many more similarities than differences between women and men. Rather than put-downs or coercion, you can positively influence your partner and be open to his positive influence with you.

Melinda and Richard had a lot of work in front of them as they planned their lives, marriage, and family. They confronted the poisons in their relationship so these no longer dominated their view of each other and the relationship. Individually and as a couple they were growing psychologically, relationally, and sexually. They were committed to replacing dramatic sex with a couple sexual style which promoted desire/pleasure/eroticism/satisfaction so that sexuality had a 15–20% role in energizing their bond.

Gender Similarities and Differences

Although there are conflicts involving gender differences in work, pay, household chores, and childcare, the most challenging involves sexuality. By its nature, sexuality is a highly personal, emotional, and complex issue whether discussing desire, function, orgasm, birth control, or monogamy. The advantage of the male—female double standard was the rules were clear; sex was the man's domain—he had greater desire, achieved spontaneous erections, and was orgasmic 100% of the time. Birth control, intimacy, and relational stability were the woman's domain. Although not acknowledged, it was expected that the man would "fool around," but the woman had to be faithful (or there would be terrible consequences). Clear, but stupid, rules with a very sexist bias.

The equity model of female—male sexuality is challenging. The equity model requires both the woman and man to confront fears and concerns. Is it okay for you to have strong sexual desire? Does this mean you'll have affairs and undermine marital stability? Will your sexual desire and response intimidate him, causing erectile dysfunction? Will you demand an orgasm each time? Can he deliver a perfect sex performance to satisfy you? Will he get a vasectomy rather than you be sterilized? What will happen to relationship attachment and security?

We are strong advocates for the equity model and strong critics of the traditional double standard. We are even stronger advocates of the woman and man being intimate and erotic friends (McCarthy & Bodnar, 2005). This sounds easy, but, in truth, requires major changes for the woman, man, couple, and culture. Good intentions are not enough. You need to devote thought, time, communication, practice, and feedback to establish and maintain an equitable emotional and sexual relationship. This means respecting and accepting each other with recognition of individual and couple vulnerabilities as well as strengths. It means building and reinforcing a genuine sense of trust that your partner will act in your best interest. When something negative occurs, he "has your back."

Sexuality is a particularly challenging issue. The traditional approach, even for the well-intentioned man who says "I care about your sexual needs—what can I do to make sex better for you," is counter-productive. Why? Because performance anxiety and self-consciousness subvert female and couple sexuality. There is nothing more anti-erotic than self-consciousness.

What promotes sexual equity? The most important guideline is to recognize female sexuality as first class, not inferior to male sexuality. Female desire/pleasure/eroticism/satisfaction is more flexible, variable, complex, and individualistic-different, not better or worse. Although orgasm is highly valued, satisfaction is much more than orgasm. You feel satisfaction when you are not orgasmic. Traditionally, male sexuality was viewed as the "norm." For adolescent and young adult males, erections were easy and spontaneous, each encounter led to intercourse, and he was orgasmic 100% of the time. His sex response was autonomous—he needed nothing from you. Few women function autonomously. Most women learn sexuality as interactive and variable, even during the romantic love/passionate sex/idealistic (limerance) phase. After the six-month—two-year limerance phase has ended, you learn to value desire which is responsive to intimacy and touch rather than spontaneous. Pleasure, eroticism, and orgasm are integral to female sexuality. Women value variable, flexible interactive sexuality rather than totally predictable intercourse and orgasm. This learning allows you as a couple to be sexual in your 50s, 60s, 70s, and 80s.

A strong argument for the value of female sexuality is that when couples stop being sexual it is almost always the man's choice—made because he has lost confidence with erection, intercourse, and orgasm. Couple sexuality based on sharing pleasure as an intimate team is a healthier model in contrast to the individual sex performance approach with intercourse as the pass–fail test. Desire is the core factor in couple sexuality. Desire focuses on sharing pleasure while integrating intimacy and eroticism. The couple model of strong, resilient desire is healthier than one based on perfect individual performance (erection for the man and orgasm for the woman).

With the equity model, both partners value desire/pleasure/eroticism/satisfaction. Rather than a competition about who is right or better, you are intimate and erotic allies. An involved, aroused partner is the best aphrodisiac. Value mutual, synchronous sexuality—both partners experience desire/pleasure/eroticism/satisfaction. In addition, affirm the value of asynchronous sexual experiences. Flexibility, variability, and pleasure are valued; drop the individual pass–fail sex performance test. The man can enjoy the woman's capacity for multi-orgasmic response as well as accepting that your sexual satisfaction is much more than orgasm. He transitions to intercourse on his first erection and values predictable sex including a single orgasm during intercourse. Male sexuality is healthier when he accepts variable, flexible sexuality for himself and your relationship. Each partner's unique sexual pattern adds spice to your relationship.

Exercise: Ending the Power Struggle by Embracing the Equity Model

This exercise involves two phases. First, confront the impact of the traditional male—female double standard which is the basis for the war between men and women. Rather than engaging in arguments, jokes, or politically correct phrases, we urge you to be personal, concrete, and specific regarding attitudes, behaviors, and feelings. Be aware of the negative effects of power struggles on each person's psychological, relational, and sexual well-being. Explore these experiences in your family, childhood, adolescence, young adulthood, and present relationship. Be honest, specific, and personal—don't hide behind abstractions.

Your negative learnings and impacts are likely to be different than your partner's. Don't minimize differences or settle for gender stereotypes. Men experience both positive and negative consequences from the double standard as do women. Be comprehensive, honest, and personal about your experiences. Process the entire range of attitudes, behaviors, and feelings. What is your take-away about gender, the double standard, sexuality, and power struggles?

The second phase of this exercise is crucial. You can't change the past; your power for change is in the present and future. What are present negative impacts of the double standard and gender wars? Be honest, specific, and personal. What are your negative attitudes, behaviors, and feelings? Even more important, how can you build equitable attitudes, behaviors, and feelings and treat each other as respectful, trusting, and intimate friends. Good intentions are important, but are not enough. You need a plan to create an equitable relationship as well as a way to implement these changes. Learning to relate as equitable allies, especially around intimacy and sexuality, is a challenge. Commit to female—male equity and be cognizant of personal and couple challenges. For example, each partner wants mutual, synchronous sexual encounters. However, the man cannot pressure you to have an orgasm each time (or insist that orgasm during intercourse is best). That is coercive, raising self-consciousness and performance anxiety. This subverts sexual pleasure and being an intimate sexual team.

Take the initiative with a focus on your sexual voice and making requests. Equitable couple sexuality is not based on you being a clone of him, catching up sexually, or having 100% predictable orgasms. Female sexuality is healthy—variable, flexible, complex, and individualistic—not inferior to male sexuality. Equitable couples develop their unique style of pleasure, eroticism, and satisfaction. Honor your sexual voice, including feelings and preferences for initiation and sexual scenarios. It is normal and healthy that some sexual encounters are better for your partner than you (and some better for you than him). Asynchronous sexual experiences are normal and part of the equity model. Asynchronous sex is healthy as long as it is not at the expense of the partner or relationship. A crucial understanding is that it is normal for 5–15% of sexual encounters to be dissatisfying or dysfunctional. When that occurs the challenge is to laugh it off (at least shrug it off) rather than fall into a blame—counter-blame trap. Turn toward your partner rather than away. Whether the sexual experience was great, good, okay, or dissatisfying, accept this and stay on the same intimate team.

Be honest with yourself and your partner about what aspects of the equity model are working and what aspects are disappointing or frustrating. For the latter, continue to dialogue and experiment so you find a way to make it work. How can you cope with difficult issues so being an equitable sexual team is not subverted? Especially important is to emphasize pleasure and responsive desire. Female sexual desire is variable, flexible, complex, and individualistic. Most important, female sexual desire is first class.

Equity and Sexuality

The female—male equity model takes thought, time, negotiation, and work. The traditional double standard is easy to understand and is taken for granted even though it's unhealthy. The equity model requires more from the woman, man, and couple including continuing to dialogue, experiment, and modify so it is functional and rewarding. You can't take sexuality for granted nor can sexuality rest on its laurels. Women, men, and couples find the equity model is a worthwhile emotional investment yielding enhanced psychological, relational, and sexual dividends.

Whether married or in a partnered relationship, for three years or 30 years, continue to grow your intimate sexual relationship. Be open to change. The role of intimacy and sexuality is to energize your bond and promote feelings of desire and desirability. Contrary to the traditional double standard of men emphasizing sex and women emphasizing intimacy, there is solid scientific evidence that in a long-term marriage, women value a vital sexual relationship and men value an affectionate, secure bond (Heiman, et al., 2011). In a healthy relationship, both partners value intimacy, pleasuring, and eroticism.

Rather than falling into a routine, predictable sexual pattern, playful touch and unpredictable scenarios enhance desire and vitality. The "empty nest" syndrome is a misnomer. The majority of women and couples report increased personal, relational, and sexual satisfaction in the "couple again" phase. Women flourish in their 50s, 60s, 70s, and 80s (Lindau, et al., 2007). A key to flourishing is touching and sexuality. In our youth-oriented, body obsessed culture, it is easy for women above age 40 (or 60) to feel negated sexually. The key to sexual desire is touch, not visual stimuli. Valuing sensual, playful, erotic, and intercourse touch is key to desire.

The female model of sexual equity and valuing variable, flexible GES is much superior to the male autonomous, sex performance model. GES and an equitable relationship facilitates flourishing with the aging of the partners and aging of the relationship. Female sexuality flourishes from your 20s to 80s.

Who We Are and the Format of This Book

Barry and Emily McCarthy are a husband—wife writing team; this is our 13th co-authored book. When we married in 1966, the male—female double standard was dominant. We were the first in our families to graduate college and were committed to living our lives in a healthier manner than our backgrounds. We wanted to create a life we could be proud of personally and relationally. However, we assumed there would be major differences sexually. We have challenged that assumption and committed to creating a satisfying, secure, and sexual marriage. We are intimate and erotic allies who value intimacy, pleasuring, and eroticism. We are not clones of each other, but approach sexuality as partners who affirm desire/pleasure/eroticism/satisfaction.

Writing this book has been challenging and enjoyable. We are pro-female, pro-male, pro-couple, and pro-sexual. We promote the 15–20% role of sexuality in individual and couple well-being whether you are 26, 46, or 76. This book is written for women, but has value for men, couples, clinicians, and the culture. We confront the harmful effects of the traditional double standard which emphasizes male—female differences and splits intimacy and eroticism. Scientifically, clinically, and personally we advocate for the female—male equity model, valuing sexual similarities, honoring sexual differences, and accepting female sexuality as first class.

We respect each other's contributions to the writing of this book. Emily's background is in speech communication, and her writing and wisdom provides a balanced, humanistic perspective. Barry's background is a professor of psychology and a clinical psychologist with a specialty in couple and sex therapy. This book is written for the public, with grounding in scientifically and clinically validated psychological, biological/medical, and social/relational information to promote healthy sexuality. Knowledge is power. We hope to empower and motivate you to embrace female and couple sexuality. In his clinical practice, Barry dealt with chronic psychological, relational, and sexual problems. If the woman (and couple) had the motivation and skills to prevent these problems or dealt with them in the acute phase, their lives would have been so much better. Prevention is the best, cheapest, and most efficacious way to address sexual issues.

We present scientifically and clinically validated information about sexuality generally and female sexuality specifically. We provide guidelines, psychosexual skill exercises, and case studies (we use composite cases with details altered to protect confidentiality) to make concepts personal and concrete. This is not meant to be read as a text book, instead each chapter is self-contained. Read chapters which are personally relevant. The material can be read for information and concepts but is best used as an interactive learning medium. Share the materials with your spouse/partner. Talking and sharing (especially the exercises) makes these concepts personal and meaningful. Implement relevant strategies, skills, and coping techniques so that sexuality has a 15–20% positive role in your life and relationship.

This book is in opposition to the heteronormative model which advocates for heterosexual marriage as the only acceptable form of sexuality. We emphasize the woman understanding and accepting her "authentic sexual self." This includes sexual orientation (lesbian, heterosexual, bi-sexual, pan-sexual, asexual). It also includes being comfortable with how you present and accept yourself as woman.

We affirm healthy female sexuality whether you are married, partnered, divorced, single, or widowed. Our messages about healthy female sexuality are relevant for women from 20 to 90. We emphasize traditional heterosexual married couples, but most of these learnings are applicable to lesbian and partnered couples.

This is a book of ideas, guidelines, and exercises; it is not a "do it yourself therapy" book. The more information, understanding, and resources, the more likely you will make "wise" sexual decisions. Knowledge is power. The psychosexual skill exercises help you assess and change attitudes, behaviors, and feelings. Seeking sex, couple, or individual therapy is a wise decision. Appendix A provides information and guidelines on how to choose a sex therapist, couple therapist, or individual therapist. Appendix B provides suggestions for further reading on female sexuality, couple sexuality, male sexuality, and relationship satisfaction.

Summary

Finding Your Sexual Voice: Celebrating Female Sexuality empowers and motivates women and couples to embrace female sexuality. We confront the traditional male—female double standard and advocate for the female—male equity model. We explore psychological, biological/medical, and social/relational factors which promote healthy sexuality and confront factors which subvert your sexuality. This is not just a book of ideas, but of psychosexual skill exercises, guidelines, and case studies to empower you to create your sexual voice as a healthy sexual woman and couple.

2

THE NEW SEXUAL MANTRA: DESIRE/PLEASURE/EROTICISM/ SATISFACTION

In the traditional approach to sexuality, the mistaken belief was that eroticism, intercourse, and orgasm was the man's domain, while intimacy, pleasuring, and satisfaction was the woman's domain. "Foreplay" involved the man stimulating the woman so that she would be ready for the "real thing"—intercourse. In the traditional view, "sex=intercourse."

There is a new mantra in the sexuality field—desire/pleasure/eroticism/ satisfaction (Foley, Kope, & Sugrue, 2012). An empowering aspect of the new mantra is that it is applicable to both women and men. Adolescent and young adult men learn that sex is easy, predictable, and in his control. Male sexual response is autonomous—he experiences desire, erection, intercourse, and orgasm needing nothing from his partner. However, this learning backfires with aging. When couples stop being sexual—whether at 40, 50, 60, or 70—it is almost always the man's decision, made unilaterally and conveyed non-verbally. He has lost confidence with erection and intercourse. For him sex involves anticipatory anxiety, performance-oriented intercourse as a pass–fail test, leading to frustration, embarrassment, and eventually avoidance (Feldman, et al., 1994). The woman feels confused, abandoned, and unsure whether to blame herself, him, or their relationship. Approximately one in three couples stop being sexual between 60–65 and two in three between 70–75. This is preventable if the man and woman had adopted the new mantra of desire/pleasure/ eroticism/satisfaction in their 50s, or ideally in their 20s.

Male sexual socialization emphasizes that a "real man is able to have sex with any woman, any time, in any situation." The assumption was that what made a man a man was spontaneous erections and perfect intercourse performance. This mistaken notion has oppressed men across generations and cultures. Men who challenge this oppressive demand are belittled as "wimps," "inadequate," or "not man enough." Few men have the awareness and courage to challenge the individual perfect sex performance myth, especially not with male peers. The psychologically healthy man shares broad-based, variable, flexible sexuality with the woman. This is especially important when both partners are committed to a satisfying, secure, and sexual relationship.

Sex as a Team Sport

The essence of couple sexuality is giving and receiving pleasure-oriented touching. Couple sexuality is a team sport, not an individual sex performance. Sexuality involves intimacy, pleasuring, and eroticism. Sex is best when the woman and man are intimate and erotic allies. Why is sex as an intimate team so hard to accept? In part, it's because as adolescents and young adults, sexual socialization was so different for women and men. The major reason is the oppressive male—female double standard. As people age, especially after 40, and in a married or partnered relationship, there are many more psychological, relational, and sexual similarities than differences between women and men. The overlearned and overvalued double standard damages the sexuality of men, women, and couples. Yet, it is difficult to change. The adolescent/young adult learning must be confronted. The couple value being intimate and erotic friends who embrace desire/pleasure/eroticism/satisfaction.

Desire

Desire is the core sexual dimension. Positive anticipation is a key to desire. You deserve sexuality which energizes your relationship. Desire is facilitated by freedom, choice, a pleasure orientation, and unpredictable sexual scenarios and techniques.

Males learn about sexual desire in a very different way than females. Sex is viewed as integral to being a man, associated with spontaneous erections, the desire for intercourse, and predictable orgasm. Most males begin masturbating between 10 and 14 and are orgasmic daily or several times a week. The typical male experiences first orgasm during couple sex between 15 and 21, whether with manual stimulation, intercourse, oral stimulation, or rubbing stimulation. Males have less fear of pregnancy, contracting an STI, and don't worry about being labeled a "slut." A sexually active male adolescent is viewed as a "stud."

These learnings work for adolescent and young adult males, although we do not believe this is a healthy learning. Certainly, it does not serve the adult male well, especially after age 40 and in a married or partnered relationship.

Rather than pretending gender stereotypes are true of all males and females, let us carefully examine positive and negative learnings about desire/pleasure/eroticism/satisfaction. Remember the crucial guideline—value psychological, relational, and sexual similarities. For adults in an intimate sexual relationship it is a myth that "Men are from Mars and Women are from Venus."

Desire is the core factor in healthy female, male, and couple sexuality. Unfortunately, women experience much higher rates of low sexual desire than men (Meana, 2010). Male sexual dysfunction, especially erectile dysfunction and ejaculatory inhibition, causes secondary low sexual desire which results in the man avoiding sex. When couples stop being sexual, whether at 35, 55, or 75, it is almost always the man's decision, made unilaterally and conveyed non-verbally. He has lost confidence with erections, intercourse, and orgasm. Sex is frustrating and embarrassing. His sexuality is controlled by anticipatory anxiety, performance anxiety focused on intercourse as a pass–fail test, and frustration which eventually leads to sexual avoidance. He says to himself: "I don't want to start something I can't finish."

The new sexual mantra emphasizes desire for pleasure-oriented touch. For adult women and men, it is touch and emotional awareness that leads to sexual desire rather than a spontaneous urge, erotic fantasy, visual stimuli, or wanting an orgasm. The new understanding, especially for women, centers on "responsive sexual desire." Unlike the traditional male model which focused on easy erection as the "natural" way to experience desire, the new sophisticated, complex, and nuanced model of "responsive sexual desire" reflects similarities between women and men and recognizes the multiple roles, opportunities, and meanings of touch and sexuality.

This new model includes psychological, biological, and social/relational factors. You can promote or subvert desire. Desire is a complex process which can and does wax and wane, but is resilient (McCarthy, 2015).

Psychological factors which facilitate desire are positive anticipation, intimacy, and touching. You deserve sex to be healthy at this time in your life and in this relationship. Desire is facilitated by choice, freedom, and unpredictability. Unfortunately, desire is easy to kill. Psychological factors that negate desire include performance pressure, coercion, fear of negative consequences, anger, anticipatory anxiety, and routine, mechanical sex. It is crucial to keep sex poisons out of the system. Even more important is to keep desire vital and resilient.

Biologically/medically, anything which is good for your physical body is good for your sexual body. In addition, behavioral health patterns of sleep, regular exercise, healthy eating, no smoking, and moderate or no drinking are crucial. In terms of negative biological factors, it is not aging which interferes with desire, but illness and the side-effects of medications (especially hypertensive and anti-depression medications). Negative behavioral health habits—poor sleep, lack of exercise, poor eating, obesity, smoking, alcohol or drug abuse—interfere with sexual function and desire (this is true for both women and men). Illness or disability does not stop sexual desire but does alter sexual function which can indirectly reduce desire.

Socially and relationally, the attitudes, values, and expectations of the partner and culture have a major impact on sexual desire. The core cultural factor is whether a satisfying, secure, and sexual relationship is valued and promoted. For example, movies seldom focus on marital sex; "hot sex" portrays pre-marital or extra-marital couples. Hot sex is new, spontaneous, dramatic, illicit, and idealized. Marital sexuality which integrates intimacy and eroticism and promotes a satisfying, secure bond is ignored. The couple turning toward each other as intimate and erotic allies is crucial for desire. Sexual desire cannot be taken for granted nor treated with benign neglect. Maintaining strong, resilient desire is both an individual responsibility and a couple challenge.

Couple therapists emphasize communication, loving feelings, intimacy, and a secure bond, with the false assumption that this automatically generates sexual desire. The challenge for couples, whether married or partnered, straight or lesbian, is to integrate intimacy and eroticism. Traditionally, there has been a gender split where men valued eroticism and women valued intimacy. This split subverts relational and sexual satisfaction. Strong, resilient sexual desire is facilitated when both partners value intimacy and eroticism.

Pleasure

The second component of the new mantra is nondemand pleasuring. This involves sensual and playful touching inside and outside the bedroom. Pleasuring is a basic dimension of sexuality whether it proceeds to intercourse or not. This is core for the broad, flexible approach to couple sexuality. Of course, pleasuring can be a path to arousal, intercourse, and orgasm. However, intercourse is not the sole or even chief function of pleasuring.

Sensuality is the foundation for sexual response and facilitates desire. Sensual touch involves non-genital massage, cuddling on the couch while watching a DVD, touching when going to sleep or on awakening, giving or receiving back or foot rubs. On a 10-point scale of subjective pleasure/arousal where "0" is neutral and "10" is orgasm, sensual touch creates sensations/feelings of "1–3."

Playful touch consists of both genital and non-genital pleasuring with receptivity to sensations involving "4–5" on the pleasure/arousal scale. Examples of playful touch include whole body massage, touching while bathing or showering together, "fooling around," romantic or erotic dancing, and playing games like strip poker or Twister. Playful touch is seductive and energizing. It has value in itself as well as a bridge to arousal, intercourse, and orgasm.

Nondemand pleasuring validates touch for both attachment and sexual desire. Touch is the major component of desire as well as promoting variable, flexible, and unpredictable scenarios. Nondemand pleasuring can have a number of roles, meanings, and outcomes.

Pleasuring (as opposed to performance) validates the importance of giving touch and being touched. Sex is not a pass–fail test of intercourse or orgasm; sexuality is a sharing of pleasure-oriented experiences which have a range of dimensions and outcomes. Pleasuring is the foundation for desire. Foreplay is a one-way experience of preparing the woman for intercourse. The foreplay approach subverts female desire. A couple pleasure-orientation of giving and receiving touch promotes desire for the woman, man, and couple.

Eroticism

Erotic scenarios and techniques are the most confusing and controversial aspect of couple sexuality. On the subjective arousal scale, erotic touch varies from "6–10." Couples usually transition to intercourse rather than continuing erotic stimulation to orgasm. Others enjoy the erotic flow of manual, oral, or rubbing stimulation and allow this to naturally result in orgasm. This pattern of erotic stimulation to orgasm is particularly important for women.

Eroticism is different than pleasuring; complementary, not oppositional. Eroticism involves taking personal and sexual risks, creativity, mystery, unpredictability, and vitality. Nondemand pleasuring is sensual and playful, warm and sharing. Eroticism is explicitly sexual, lustful, and involves intense feelings and sensations, resulting in high arousal, erotic flow, and orgasm. Eroticism typically flows to intercourse, but that is not a demand.

Eroticism involves three arousal styles:

1. Partner interaction arousal.
2. Self-entrancement arousal.
3. Role enactment arousal.

These are three very different ways of experiencing eroticism but can be complementary (Mosher, 1980).

Partner interaction arousal is the most common pattern, involving giving and receiving erotic stimulation. It is the arousal pattern seen in R-rated movies and the erotic extension of the "give to get" pleasuring guideline. Each partner's arousal plays off the other's. Partner interaction arousal is illustrated by the adage "an aroused partner is the major aphrodisiac." Some couples only use partner interaction arousal, while others also utilize self-entrancement and/or role enactment arousal.

The second most frequent pattern is self-entrancement arousal. The key to self-entrancement arousal is taking turns—one partner is the giver, the other the receiver—taking in erotic feelings and sensations. Self-entrancement arousal is very different than foreplay. The receiving partner is mindful and actively involved in the arousal/eroticism process. Many couples, especially with aging, utilize self-entrancement arousal on a regular basis.

Self-entrancement arousal emphasizes the receiver being relaxed, open to and mindful of erotic feelings, taking in pleasure, enjoying erotic sensations, including the freedom to let go and invite erotic flow to orgasm.

Some couples switch roles during an erotic encounter, others transition to intercourse at high levels of erotic flow, and still others enjoy an erotic, asynchronous experience. Self-entrancement arousal is positive for the giving partner even though less erotically intense. Self-entrancement arousal confronts the "tyranny of mutuality"—not all sex has to be serious, intimate, and mutual. Self-entrancement arousal is an integral component of couple sexuality.

Role enactment arousal receives by far the most attention in sexuality books and on internet sex sites. Role enactment arousal brings something external into the couple sexual repertoire. This can involve sex toys (blindfold, vibrator, paddle, dildo, handcuffs), X-rated videos, playing out an erotic fantasy, being sexual in front of a mirror or taping a sexual scenario, using fetish material, or being sexual when cross-dressed. The couple sexual style most amenable to role enactment arousal is the Emotionally Expressive sexual style. The two sexual styles where it is not a good fit are the Traditional and Best Friend styles. (We discuss couple sexual styles in Chapter 10.)

Role enactment arousal can enhance the couple sexual repertoire. It spices up the relationship and adds an unpredictable, vital dimension.

However, we have a real concern that the manner in which role enactment arousal is promoted can intimidate rather than empower the couple. For example, traditional porn videos can serve as a bridge to sexual desire or provide an erotic charge. Porn works best when both partners recognize that erotic fantasy is very different than real-life couple sex. Erotic fantasies and scenarios are sexually charged because they are so different than real-life sexuality. In the great majority of cases, what works as an erotic fantasy is totally different than couple sexuality. Playing out an erotic fantasy is more likely to result in a sexual "dud" than a highly erotic sexual experience (and rob the fantasy of its sexual charge).

The message of porn is that the crazier the scenario and the crazier the woman the more erotic she is. Many women disown eroticism. She distrusts eroticism whether on video or the internet. She fears this is what her partner really wants, and she can never measure up to this crazy sex ideal. What is the reality? Erotic fantasies, images, videos, and scenarios are all about fantasy, not about what the man wants from a real-life woman with whom he has an intimate relationship. It is worth repeating, erotic fantasies/videos are a totally different dimension than real-life couple sex. It is an "apples—oranges" comparison which has no real importance for couple sexuality.

What is the essence of eroticism and what is its importance? Integrated eroticism is an integral dimension of healthy female and couple sexuality. Eroticism allows you to experience arousal, erotic flow, intercourse, and orgasm. Sexual pleasure flows to eroticism and orgasm whether using partner interaction arousal, self-entrancement arousal, or role enactment arousal. Eroticism enhances sexual vitality and energizes your bond.

Satisfaction

Does "orgasm=satisfaction"? No, satisfaction is much more than orgasm, and yes you can have a satisfying sexual experience even when one or both partners are not orgasmic.

The essence of satisfaction is reinforcing positive feelings about you as a sexual woman as well as feeling bonded and energized as a couple. Orgasm is an integral component of female, male, and couple sexuality.

However, orgasm as a pass–fail individual performance test subverts sexual satisfaction. Pleasure, eroticism, and orgasm are positive, integral components which enhance satisfaction.

Satisfaction is a complex phenomenon involving cognitive, behavioral, physical, emotional, and value components. Satisfaction involves a range of dimensions—from highly satisfying to good and okay. It is possible to be orgasmic yet feel alienated. More commonly, you are not orgasmic yet feel emotionally bonded. In fact, sometimes the sexual experience is more satisfying for the non-orgasmic partner than the orgasmic partner.

An often-neglected component of sexuality is afterplay. Afterplay is integral to couple sexuality and facilitates satisfaction. You have just shared an intense sexual experience; satisfaction is enhanced if you share an involved afterplay experience.

The most common afterplay scenario is warm and cuddly, but there are a range of possible emotions and scenarios. Afterplay can be playful or silly, intimate or serious, verbal or non-verbal, involve a glass of wine or a treat, lying together or sitting up, reminiscing or your own unique way of validating being a couple.

Should afterplay be a prelude to a second sexual encounter? Yes, but only if both partners are open to an erotic or intercourse scenario. One reason women avoid afterplay is the fear it will be misinterpreted as a sexual initiation. The great majority of afterplay experiences are to share, bond, and enhance satisfaction, not a second sexual encounter.

Is sex sometimes better for one partner than the other? Not only is that normal, it is true for the majority of sexual encounters. Almost all couples prefer mutual, synchronous sex where both experience desire/pleasure/eroticism/satisfaction. Among happily married, sexually functional couples the ideal scenario occurs 35–45% of the time. This does not mean that the sex wasn't satisfying (85–95% are positive). It means that it wasn't synchronous (equal). A key to sexual satisfaction is awareness that it is normal and healthy for sex to have different roles and meanings for each partner (including in the same encounter). The foundation for sexual satisfaction is positive, realistic sexual expectations. Often, there are differences in psychological, physical, and relational satisfaction—that too is normal and healthy.

Exercise: Implementing the New Mantra

This exercise asks you to make personal and concrete the mantra of desire/pleasure/eroticism/satisfaction. It involves both individual and couple components. Whether your relationship has existed for one year or 40 years, each person recalls when each sexual dimension was the most positive. Many women find that it is different for each dimension. As well, the partner often has a different remembrance of the best sexual experiences. For example, people remember desire being highest in the first few months, pleasuring best in the present, eroticism best when on vacation, and satisfaction best when you're feeling sexually understood and accepted.

Be specific and concrete—share attitudes and feelings. Some people find it easier to write about sexuality and others to speak about sexuality. The important thing is to own your experiences and share these, so your partner "gets" you and understands what you value and what makes a sexual experience satisfying for you. This exercise requires emotional courage to be transparent and vulnerable. Don't be vague, shy, or inhibited. Allow yourself to be sexually known by your partner. This enhances trust in yourself, your partner, and your sexual relationship. It is especially important if your sexual feelings and preferences are atypical or "socially unacceptable."

One of the most interesting and challenging aspects of being a sex therapist is hearing the wide range of people's feelings about sexual experiences. Let us consider examples from the pleasuring dimension. Common scenarios include taking a bath and having a glass of wine, using a lotion to enhance body massage, mutual body rub while listening to your favorite hip-hop tape. Examples of atypical pleasuring experiences include being on a nude beach and people admiring your bodies as you seductively play with each other; going to a sex-themed motel where there are ceiling mirrors; engaging in touching at 2 am under the Christmas tree; "making out" for an hour in a car parked by the lake as the sun rises.

Identifying special experiences is not a matter of "right—wrong" or proving something to your partner. Be open and genuinely share sexual feelings and experiences. When did you most value desire, pleasure, eroticism, and experience the highest level of satisfaction? Perhaps the most valuable learning is that the dimensions were experienced at different times and in different ways. A critical learning is that your partner's experiences and what he values are different than yours. Sexuality is complex and individualistic. You are not clones of each other. This is motivating and empowering.

The second part of this exercise is even more important. What are your goals for the present and future to enhance desire/pleasure/eroticism/satisfaction? Do not set romantic Hollywood goals or crazy porn goals. Set positive, realistic goals which you are personally committed to. Let's explore common and atypical desire goals. A common desire goal is to increase the frequency of sensual and playful touching with the hope that these become a bridge to desire. For you is touch (nondemand pleasuring) the key for sexual desire? Do you engage in nondemand pleasuring for itself? Are you open to pleasuring being a bridge to intercourse?

What strategies and techniques work in your sex life? Find desire sources which fit you.

Let's explore atypical sources for sexual desire. An example is planning a special erotic date. This includes asking your partner to watch the children in the afternoon so you can go for a pedicure or a massage. Afterward, instead of going home, do something you enjoy whether a swim, kayaking, shoe shopping, meeting a girlfriend for a drink, reading an erotic novel.

Instead of the usual dinner, movie, and home for sex, do something different. Rent a hotel room from 7–10 with sex before and/or after dinner. Go dancing or listen to music and be sexual in the car in a safe, secluded place. Go to a sex store and purchase a sex toy to use at home after dropping off the babysitter. These scenarios elicit desire for some couples while others find only one does (with other scenarios a turnoff). Couples create very different desire scenarios.

Create scenarios and techniques to promote vibrant, satisfying couple sexuality that has a 15–20% role in your life and relationship.

Arousal, Intercourse, and Orgasm

Women find exploring pleasuring of interest, but come back to a basic question: What about arousal, intercourse, and orgasm? Isn't that the essence of sexuality? Are desire/pleasure/eroticism/satisfaction just the politically correct words? Doesn't it all come down to whether sex works or not (meaning old-fashioned arousal, intercourse, and orgasm)?

Let us be clear—we are absolutely in favor of arousal, intercourse, and orgasm. And, yes, most sexual experiences involve those components. But, no, this is not the essence of couple sexuality. Couples have functional sex, but it does not energize their bond or promote desire. The new sexual mantra with a special focus on desire and satisfaction is motivating and empowering. Pleasuring can transition to arousal, intercourse, and orgasm. Yet, nondemand pleasuring has value in itself. Erotic scenarios are energizing, including when it does not lead to intercourse. Asynchronous (including one-way) eroticism enhances desire and satisfaction.

Let us take a different perspective. Mutual, synchronous sexual experiences involving arousal, intercourse, and orgasm are highly valued. However, if that is the only acceptable sex it will subvert desire. By its nature, couple sexuality is variable and flexible, with a number of roles, meanings, and outcomes. Healthy couple sexuality is much more than arousal, intercourse, and orgasm (Frank, Anderson, & Rubinstein, 1978).

Rebecca and James

Rebecca and James were a religiously and socially conservative couple in a 31-year marriage. For the first time in 30 years they were a "couple again" after launching their last child into college. For most couples, the "empty nest" syndrome is a misnomer. The majority of couples find the "couple again" phase an impetus for personal, relational, and sexual growth. For most couples, sexual satisfaction goes down at the birth of a first child and does not go up again until the last child leaves home. This does not mean that Rebecca regretted having three children. Although reducing opportunities for personal, couple, and sexual time, Rebecca and James enjoyed parenting and were proud of their five-person family.

In the couple again phase, they had an opportunity to embrace desire/pleasure/eroticism/satisfaction after 31 years of marriage. Like many couples in their 50s, they had fallen into the pattern of being sexual once a week, usually late on a weekend night. Sex was functional but not vibrant or satisfying. The sexual encounter was a routine of five minutes of foreplay, four minutes of intercourse, and two—three minutes of afterplay. Functional, but not special or energizing.

Rebecca lobbied James to come to a session with her individual therapist with the hope of starting couple therapy. James agreed to meet Rebecca's therapist (he wanted to see who she was as well as give the therapist a better idea of who he was). The therapist told Rebecca that meeting James was worthwhile—he was much different than the image the therapist had of a "closed down" man.

James suggested he and Rebecca give a six-month good faith effort to enhance couple intimacy and sexuality on their own. If that was not helpful, he was open to couple therapy with the goal of enhancing sexuality. One effect of that consultation was that the therapist refocused on Rebecca's individual issues. The therapist encouraged Rebecca to value James, the marriage, and sexuality. The trap for women in individual therapy is to blame the husband and marriage for most, if not all, problems rather than focus on her individual issues and growth.

Rebecca and James were committed to improving their lives and relationship. Rebecca missed feeling desired. James had ignored these issues because he worried about not having spontaneous erections. He was so concerned about a humiliating intercourse failure that he'd ignored Rebecca's feelings. Rather than enjoying the pleasuring/eroticism process, James rushed intercourse because he feared losing his erection. Previously, they had a predictable sexual pattern of her being orgasmic during intercourse utilizing multiple stimulation, especially manual clitoral stimulation with his or her fingers. With the rush to intercourse and worry about James' arousal/erection, sex was less fun. Rebecca was orgasmic less than a third of the time. Rebecca asking "what's wrong" made the situation even more tense and performance-oriented. Although erectile failures were infrequent, fear hung over their sexual relationship. No one was having fun sexually.

Unknown to Rebecca, James had consulted their internist to obtain a Viagra prescription with the hope that this would ensure reliable erections. When James was subjectively aroused and in an erotic flow, Viagra did result in a firm erection. However, he subverted the positive Viagra vascular effect by rushing to intercourse at low levels of arousal. Negative motivation (fear of erectile dysfunction or female non-orgasmic response) subverts sexuality.

Rebecca valued intimacy and nondemand pleasuring. However, James worried this would decrease sexual frequency and increase erectile anxiety—a fear that was not verbalized and which Rebecca was unaware of. This is a common dilemma for couples regardless of age.

Rather than falling into the traditional male—female power struggle over intercourse, Rebecca made a very insightful suggestion. Each person would commit to reading the same material (a short article) about desire/pleasure/eroticism/satisfaction. Then they shared feelings about growing their intimate sexual relationship. This reading and discussion helped James and Rebecca speak the same language about intimacy, pleasuring, and eroticism.

They made a commitment to rebuild sexual desire. They increased sexual anticipation, felt they deserved to enjoy sexuality at this time in their marriage, took advantage of the freedom of when and how to be sexual, and reduced performance pressure of erection and intercourse. They wanted to put fun, pleasure, eroticism, and unpredictability into their sexual relationship. Like most couples, James and Rebecca valued spontaneous sex. And like most couples, the reality is that most sexual encounters are planned or semi-planned. James turned toward Rebecca as his intimate sexual ally rather than feel he had to perform for her. Adopting this mindset enhances sexual anticipation.

Nondemand pleasuring did not include a prohibition on intercourse but did involve a commitment to not rush to intercourse. They agreed Rebecca would initiate the transition to intercourse when she felt high subjective arousal. James was open to multiple stimulation during intercourse to increase erotic flow. Rebecca especially liked giving and receiving stimulation. She valued clitoral stimulation, and he valued receiving testicle stimulation. The sexual encounter, including intercourse, was vital and engaging. Enjoying pleasuring and erotic flow made orgasm more satisfying.

Traditionally, afterplay had been routine and short. Now afterplay was involving and meaningful. Sometimes it was warm and cuddly, other times fun and silly, and occasionally intimate and bonding. Not all sexual encounters were satisfying, but the vibrancy of their desire/pleasure/eroticism/satisfaction was markedly improved. Rebecca and James were committed to being a sexual couple in their 60s, 70s, and 80s.

Summary

The new mantra of desire/pleasure/eroticism/satisfaction is valuable for women, men, and couples. It facilitates speaking a common language about sexual feelings and scenarios as well as the roles and meanings of sexuality. Especially important is the recognition of female—male sexual equity. Although not clones of each other, both partners value desire/pleasure/eroticism/satisfaction. Accept that desire is the core dimension of sexuality and is best approached as a couple issue. Sexual function involving arousal, intercourse, and orgasm is very important, but satisfaction is more important. You want to feel good about yourself as a sexual woman and you as an intimate sexual couple.

3

FIRST-CLASS FEMALE SEXUALITY

A core concept is that female sexuality is first class, not inferior to male sexuality. Traditionally, both mental health professionals and the public assumed the "common sense" belief that male sexuality was stronger and more natural. Biological/medical professionals explained this by testosterone, psychological professionals emphasized that sex was an integral component of masculinity, and sociologists emphasized gender differences—men had more freedom to be sexual. Female social socialization emphasized negative sexual health and relational consequences. Adolescent and young adult men got spontaneous erections and experienced autonomous sexual response while the woman had to "catch up."

In adult relationships, especially marriage (or a life partnership) there are many more similarities than differences between women and men. Couples who embrace the equity model of a female—male intimate relationship enjoy enhanced sexual desire and satisfaction. Unfortunately, the culture has not caught up with the new concepts and science. The adolescent approach to sex subverts adult female and couple sexuality.

Female sexuality is more variable, flexible, complex, and individualistic than male sexuality, but not inferior (McCarthy & Wald, 2016). The female experience of responsive sexual desire; valuing nondemand pleasuring; embracing sensual, playful, and erotic touch as valuable for themselves; accepting that satisfaction is more than orgasm; and embracing variable, flexible sexual scenarios sets the stage for healthy sexuality in your 40s, 50s, 60s, 70s, and 80s. When couples stop being sexual it is almost always the man's choice made because he has lost confidence with erection, intercourse, and orgasm. The "natural" male model of spontaneous erection, each encounter proceeding to intercourse, and one predictable ejaculation is neither healthy nor first class. The variable, flexible Good Enough Sex (GES) model of couple sexuality which emphasizes sharing pleasure is much superior for the woman, man, couple, and culture. The rigid individual sex performance model of intercourse and orgasm as a pass–fail test is a major cause of sex dysfunction and low sex frequency. The female model of intimate, interactive couple sexuality focused on giving and receiving pleasure-oriented touching; acceptance of the range of roles, meanings, and outcomes of sexuality; valuing desire and satisfaction as more important than orgasm; and a commitment to desire/pleasure/eroticism/satisfaction rather than perfect individual sex performance is healthier (Nagoski, 2015). This model results in first-class sexuality for women and men. It honors complexity and confronts sexual perfectionism. By its nature, couple sexuality is variable, flexible, and has a range of meanings rather than being a pass–fail individual sex test.

Giving and receiving pleasure-oriented touch is the core of female desire and responsivity. This is in stark contrast to traditional "foreplay." The foreplay approach, even with a loving, well-intentioned partner, can squelch your desire/pleasure/eroticism/satisfaction. In foreplay, you are passive while the man tries to turn you on so you are ready for intercourse. There are so many things wrong with the traditional foreplay scenario, but the worst is the passive role. Sexuality is an involved, active process. During self-entrancement arousal (taking turns receiving and giving touching), you are active and mindful in the receiving role. You are in charge of the transition from sensual/playful touch to erotic stimulation. Most women are not receptive to erotic stimulation until subjective arousal is in the 4–5 range. Focused genital stimulation at low levels of subjective arousal causes self-consciousness which is anti-erotic. This is what happens in foreplay. Rather than enjoying the pleasuring/eroticism process, you feel you're taking too long or worry he's becoming bored. These cognitive and emotional distractions subvert pleasure and sexual responsivity. Often, your partner is well-intentioned and has read a bestselling book or blog about how to stimulate women to ensure you are turned-on and orgasmic. Don't get into a power struggle nor put him down as "sexually stupid." Assure him you can enjoy being sexual and need him as your intimate and erotic ally. Pleasuring is about you being active and involved, not passive or working to speed up your arousal. Understanding the distinction between being responsible for your pleasure and traditional "foreplay" is crucial for healthy female sexuality.

You are in charge of your desire/pleasure/eroticism/satisfaction. It is not his responsibility to produce desire or orgasm for you. The key is the integration of personal responsibility for sex and being an intimate sexual team. Don't treat this as a "politically correct" slogan nor an isolated cognitive understanding. It is a cognitive-behavioral-emotional commitment to being a healthy sexual woman who takes responsibility for your sexuality. Accept pleasure and remain mindful of your responsibility for sexuality.

Exercise: First-Class Female Sexuality

To make these concepts personal and concrete we encourage you to design and play out a first-class sexual scenario.

Start by establishing the conditions and milieu which invite a sexual experience. This is not about a perfect romantic setting or a powerful erotic charge, but about positive, realistic personal and situational factors which enhance your sexual anticipation. For some the important factor is being well-rested, for others it is reading a sexy passage or watching an R-rated movie, an erotic fantasy about a stranger or sexy co-worker, going for a bike ride and showering before sex, sex after a gourmet meal and two glasses of wine, feeling close and loving, celebrating a personal or family accomplishment, cuddling on the couch watching your favorite romantic comedy, sex as a refuge after a stressful day at work, sex after a relaxing bath. What are your conditions which invite a first-class sexual experience, creating positive anticipation and a sense of deserving pleasure?

What milieu/environmental factors invite first-class sexuality? Stay away from unrealistic scenarios like a $2000 hotel suite overlooking the ocean. Features could include privacy, comfort, inviting space, sense of security, a fire in the fireplace or a scented candle, dimmed lighting, jazz or romantic music in the background. What milieu facilitates your receptivity/responsivity for a sexual encounter?

What is your preferred initiation scenario? Do you enjoy initiating? If so, verbal or non-verbal? Playful or direct? Or do you prefer that he initiates? Do you want him to be seductive, erotic, or say he needs you? Don't worry about it being socially acceptable. What type of initiation feels inviting for you?

What is your favorite way to begin the sexual encounter? Do you like a seductive beginning; sensual touching, kissing, or scratching your back; playful touch; direct genital stimulation; a lustful "I need you now"; "making-out"; a slow build-up?

For nondemand pleasuring do you prefer give-and-take touching, being the receptive partner, the giving partner, using a lotion, proceeding from non-genital to genital touching, mixing genital and non-genital pleasuring?

What is your favorite way of transitioning from pleasuring to eroticism? Most women are not receptive/responsive to erotic stimulation until subjective arousal is a 4 or 5. What is your pattern? Do you enjoy starting eroticism with breast stimulation, vulva stimulation, clitoral stimulation, or multiple stimulation? Do you give yourself permission to use erotic fantasies as a bridge to erotic flow? Do you prefer giving and receiving (partner interaction arousal) or taking turns (self-entrancement arousal)? Do you utilize sexual toys or play erotic games (role enactment arousal)?

What is your "orgasmic voice"? Do you prefer manual, intercourse, oral, rubbing, or vibrator stimulation to orgasm? Is your pattern to be orgasmic before intercourse, during intercourse, or in afterplay? Is multiple stimulation or a single, focused stimulation your preferred technique for orgasm? Is your orgasmic pattern 90% of encounters, 70%, 50%, or a different pattern? Orgasm is a positive, integral dimension of female sexuality. Rather than the performance pressure of the "perfect" or "right" orgasm, accept your "orgasmic voice" pattern(s). Few women have the same orgasmic pattern as men—a predictable single orgasm during intercourse with no additional stimulation. Orgasm is about acceptance, not proving something to your partner or living up to a performance goal (based on a myth). Female orgasmic response is variable, flexible, individualistic, first class, and not inferior to male orgasm.

What is your preferred approach to intercourse? Remember, one in three women are never (or almost never) orgasmic during intercourse. Orgasm with erotic stimulation is normal and healthy, not a dysfunction. Of the two in three women who are orgasmic during intercourse, the key is multiple stimulation. Intercourse is a natural continuation of the pleasuring/eroticism process, not a pass–fail test. Most women prefer to transition to intercourse at high levels of erotic flow, 7–8, rather than beginning arousal of 4–5. Other women enjoy a quick transition to intercourse. What is your preference of when to transition, which partner initiates intercourse, and who guides intromission? What is your favorite intercourse position—man on top, woman on top, side to side, sitting/kneeling, rear entry? Do you enjoy intercourse as an involving experience or do you prefer intense, hard-driving intercourse? Do you like to stay with one intercourse position or switch positions? Do you have particularly appealing intercourse techniques or variations? What kind of intercourse thrusting is best for you—rapid, in-out, long, slow, up-down, circular thrusting?

What type of afterplay scenarios promote satisfaction? Do you prefer a warm scenario, a playful scenario, an action-oriented scenario like showering together, a cup of tea or glass of wine, planning a couple trip, recalling a meaningful emotional time, playing a word game, playful touch and starting again? Afterplay has a range of roles and meanings, adding to bonding and satisfaction. Afterplay is integral to first-class sexuality.

> As you review your preferences and choices, can you create one, two, or three first-class sexual scenarios? By its nature couple sexuality is variable, flexible, and has a range of roles, meanings, and outcomes. Embrace first-class female and couple sexuality.

Dealing with Mediocre, Dissatisfying, or Dysfunctional Experiences

Celebrating first-class sexuality includes acceptance of occasional mediocre, dissatisfying, or dysfunctional encounters. Among happily married, sexually satisfied couples, 5–15% of sexual experiences are dissatisfying or dysfunctional. This is an important reality. Turning toward each other rather than apologizing or blaming is integral to healthy sexuality. Sometimes the message of sex dysfunction is a need to address a problem, but most often this is a normal "blip" that is calmly accepted. Be sexual in the next few days when you feel aware, awake, and open to desire/pleasure/eroticism/satisfaction. First-class sexuality involves positive anticipation, pleasure-oriented sexuality, and a regular rhythm of sexual connection. Do not be afraid of or overreact to occasional mediocre, dissatisfying, or dysfunctional encounters. You are a human being, not a perfectly functioning machine. First-class female sexuality accepts the range of sexual feelings, roles, meanings, and outcomes. You are not burdened by the traditional male pass–fail performance orientation.

Even dysfunctional sex can have a "silver lining." It allows you to value vibrant, satisfying sex as well as keeps you human rather than arrogant. The media and movies do not accept mediocre or dysfunctional sex. Sexual problems are treated as a sign of a fatally flawed relationship. In truth, a sign of a healthy sexual relationship is the ability to accept occasional dissatisfying or dysfunctional sex and turn toward each other rather than avoid or blame. Even the best sexual couple will experience a negative sexual encounter at least once a year (even once a month).

Gloria and Sam

Neither Gloria nor Sam grew up with a model of healthy female sexuality. Thirty-eight-year-old Gloria was a well-educated woman who had learned important lessons from the feminist movement. In college she'd taken a women's studies course which emphasized pregnancy prevention, rape, sexual abuse, and HIV/STI. All of these are important, but do not address healthy female sexuality. Gloria did not have a personal model of first-class sexuality.

Gloria was 29 when she met 31-year-old Sam. He was a solid boyfriend who was upfront about not believing in marriage. Sam treated Gloria well and was an involved, caring lover, but they did not discuss a long-term commitment. They put more energy into their careers than their relational lives. Gloria had the opportunity to buy a two-bedroom townhouse in the city. Sam encouraged her to take the financial risk and agreed he would help by paying rent. Gloria was proud of her new home and enjoyed personalizing and decorating it. She valued Sam's input and help, but it was her place.

They celebrated their first year at the townhouse by Sam cooking a gourmet meal. Afterward, they had an intense sexual encounter. Lying in bed, Sam said this was the best time in his life—they were a great couple, thriving in their careers, had good friends, and enjoyed a lovely house. Sam asked Gloria if she would go with him to visit his family who lived 1000 miles away. Gloria was touched and said that was a great idea. Sam had met Gloria's parents who lived in the metro area.

On the visit, her future mother-in-law took Gloria aside and told her she was the first woman Sam had brought home—a real surprise for Gloria. She certainly had loving and sexual feelings for Sam, but her assumption was that this was not a potential life partnership. Sam's parents divorced when he was 9. It was and continues to this day to be a bitter divorce. His father married and divorced twice more—Sam had a number of half-siblings with whom he had a distant relationship. His father lived in a different state with a woman who had five children. Sam exchanged texts with his father on birthdays, Christmas, and Father's Day, but it was a marginal relationship. In contrast, Sam was close to his mother and brother. The brother drove with his wife and child to meet Gloria. She realized this was a complicated family, as most are, but liked the mother, and especially the brother's wife and child. On the drive home, Sam said his family was made up of good people, but he wanted a better quality of life in terms of career, finances, and living situation. Gloria agreed and noted that she and Sam had a good life.

It was Sam who introduced the topic of their emotional and sexual relationship. This was the healthiest relationship he'd ever been in, but feared they could not maintain this level of relational satisfaction. Gloria was not a romantic idealist, but believed that aware, motivated couples can have a satisfying, secure, and sexual marriage. Her optimism allowed Sam to question his assumptions about relational and sexual realities. The most important thing Gloria said was that she felt they had a first-class relationship, and she wouldn't settle for a dissatisfying or mediocre relationship. This confronted a basic belief of Sam's—women wanted marriage and children as a goal for itself. Yes, Gloria would like marriage and children, but no that was not her core goal. She wanted a satisfying relationship which was secure and sexual. She was not willing to settle for a marginal relationship or non-sexual marriage for the sake of a family.

Gloria and Sam explored what a first-class emotional and sexual marriage would mean for them. Confronting attitudes and emotions directly is crucial for problem-solving. Gloria and Sam agreed they wanted their lives to be healthier than what they had experienced growing up, especially sexually.

Both Gloria and Sam had experienced the sexual roller coaster of dating relationships. Sam had been disappointed that after the limerance phase, sex felt more like a minefield than a pleasure. After the romantic love/passionate sex phase, Sam and previous girlfriends were not able to create a couple sexual style. The sexual relationship became a source of conflict. Gloria's experience was somewhat different. She too experienced the dating sexual roller coaster. The quality of the relationship depended on her desire to remain emotionally engaged with the boyfriend.

Gloria wanted a first-class sexual relationship where desire/pleasure/ eroticism/satisfaction remained vital. She and Sam would be intimate and erotic allies through good and bad times. She was committed to creating a couple sexual style with strong, resilient sexual desire. This was a new understanding for Sam. They were aware that sexuality was not the most important factor in a relationship. They did value the role of sexuality in energizing their bond and keeping it special. Sam's desire for Gloria was genuine. This was his opportunity for a satisfying, secure, and sexual marriage.

Of all the decisions people make in life—career, where to live, who to marry—the hardest decision to change is having children. It's easier to change houses, careers, marriage than it is to leave a child. Gloria was thrilled to learn Sam was pro-child. She envisioned having two children within a secure marriage. Because of the age factor they could not follow the guideline of waiting two years after marriage to conceive a child. She was committed to beating the odds and maintaining a first-class marriage and sexual relationship while parenting.

Gloria and Sam realized that marriage is very different than cohabitation. In their first two years of marriage they created a bond of respect, trust, and emotional commitment; adopted the Complementary couple sexual style; maintained strong, resilient sexual desire; remained intimate and erotic friends; and attended prepared childbirth classes. It was not easy, but very worthwhile in creating a first-class marriage, sexuality, and family. They were proud of their lives but would not take their relationship for granted. Sexuality continues to have a 15–20% role of energizing their bond and promoting feelings of desire and desirability. Gloria and Sam were committed to desire/pleasure/eroticism/satisfaction during their parenting years.

An Important Dialogue about First-Class Sexuality: Fidelity and Monogamy

Traditionally, couples assumed their relationship would be monogamous. This is an unhealthy assumption whether the couple's values are traditional or non-traditional. We urge you to make a clear emotional agreement about what you value about your relationship (fidelity) and your emotional and sexual boundaries (monogamy). Approximately 35–45% of American marriages involve some type of extra-marital affair (EMA)

(Baucom, et al., 2017). EMAs are an example of behavior being multi-causal, multi-dimensional, with large individual, couple, cultural, and value differences. EMAs can be in person or on-line, paid or choice, involve intercourse or erotic sexuality, be a love affair or a high opportunity/low involvement encounter. EMAs have different meanings for the involved vs. injured partner. The majority of marriages survive EMAs. The most common EMA is a male high opportunity/low involvement EMA (which is the easiest to recover from). The most challenging EMA is the female comparison EMA because it involves a combination of emotional and sexual factors and is a reversal of the double standard.

Contrary to traditional assumptions, a healthy marriage and sex life does not protect against an EMA. The most common cause of an EMA is high opportunity. Certain jobs have a high EMA rate—including "road warriors" (whether white or blue collar). Certain issues (alcoholism or insecurity) make the couple particularly vulnerable. Also, contrary to "common sense," EMAs are most likely to occur early in the marriage. Cohabitating couples have higher rates of EMA than dating or married couples (Allen, et al., 2005).

This information is not meant to intimate or scare you, but to motivate you to make a clear, genuine agreement about EMAs with your spouse/partner. Do not assume. What does relational fidelity mean to each of you? Traditionally, it meant a commitment to prioritizing the couple relationship in good and bad times and not having major secrets. Marriage meets needs for intimacy and security better than any other relationship. Does fidelity mean a first-class satisfying, secure, and sexual relationship? Or does fidelity mean children and family? We advocate for satisfying and secure relationships, but these are separate dimensions. There are highly satisfying sexual relationships which are vulnerable and not resilient when facing hard times. On the other extreme, spouse abuse and alcoholic marriages are very stable—divorce rates go up when alcoholism and spouse abuse ends.

In part, this is caused by the couple not being aware that it will take three to six months to learn to be sexual in a sober or non-violent milieu.

Don't be "politically correct" and don't assume. What do you value about relational fidelity and what does he value? Love and good intentions are crucial, but not enough. You need to reach a clear, serious commitment of what you value and what fidelity means to you personally and relationally.

Perhaps 80–85% of couples (especially married couples) affirm monogamy. It is crucial to be clear and specific about what monogamy entails and what monogamy boundaries are. Monogamy is not driven by fear, jealousy, hyper vigilance, or a "holier than thou" attitude. Monogamy is a positive emotional commitment to satisfying couple sexuality and honoring the trust/intimacy bond. The majority of married women and men masturbate—is that acceptable? The majority of married woman and men utilize private erotic fantasy (not verbalized or played out)—is that acceptable? Is use of porn or erotic materials acceptable? Is flirting in person or on-line acceptable? Is having a "romantic crush" acceptable? Be clear and specific about what is valued and what is not acceptable.

A motivating strategy for traditional couples is an emotional agreement to prevent EMA. There are three components to this agreement:

1. Be aware of your personal vulnerabilities for an EMA in terms of mood, type of person, and situation. Share these vulnerabilities with your spouse/partner. You will be surprised to learn that his vulnerabilities are quite different than yours.
2. If you are in a high-risk situation, share this with your partner rather than being guilty or secretive. The decision about an EMA is like any other life decision (moving houses, having a second child, changing careers). Discuss its impact on you, your partner, and your relationship. Make the right decision for you and your relationship.
3. If there is an EMA incident (emotional or sexual, in person or on-line) share it within 72 hours. The cover-up has more impact on trust and feelings of betrayal than the EMA itself.

If you are among the 5–15% of couples with non-traditional monogamy values, it is even more important to have a specific agreement. There are three components in the non-traditional agreement:

1. What do you value about your partner and relationship? What is the core fidelity agreement both of you are committed to?

2. What kinds of consensual non-monogamy are acceptable? Examples include triadic sex, sexual friendships (open relationships) when the spouse is gone for a month or you are a thousand miles from home, sexual play on the internet, swinging with other couples.
3. What kinds of EMAs cross a red line? Examples include falling in love, being sexual with the next-door neighbor or spouse's best friend, using the EMA to avoid couple sex, becoming pregnant or contracting an STI.

These emotional agreements/commitments recognize personal autonomy but confront secrets which are destructive for the partner and relationship. "Cheating" can and does occur with couples who agree to consensual non-monogamy.

Make an agreement which promotes personal goals for your non-traditional relationship so that consensual non-monogamy works for you.

Being a First-Class Couple and Enjoying First-Class Sexuality

You want couple sexuality which is worth having and contributes 15–20% to relational satisfaction. First-class female and couple sexuality recognizes the Good Enough Sex (GES) model as the right fit for variable, flexible couple sexuality. The perfect individual sex performance model is the antithesis of first-class sexuality. Accepting each partner's strengths and vulnerabilities is part of a first-class relationship. Couple sexuality has a range of roles, meanings, and outcomes. What makes female sexuality first class is acceptance of the desire/pleasure/eroticism/satisfaction mantra with its focus on positive, realistic expectations for your life and relationship. First-class female sexuality is about acceptance, not perfectionism. You and your partner are intimate and erotic allies. Develop a couple sexual style which balances intimacy and eroticism. Value your sexual voice and trust you are an intimate sexual team. Female sexuality is not in competition with male sexuality—rather, you embrace psychological, relational, and sexual similarities while honoring differences. First-class sexuality accepts great sex, good sex, good enough sex, mediocre sex, and occasional dysfunctional or dissatisfying sex. The key to healthy sexuality is giving and receiving pleasure-oriented touch. First-class female sexuality includes arousal, intercourse, and orgasm, but is much more than sex function. It is about sensual, playful, and erotic touch in addition to intercourse. It is about turning toward your partner whether to celebrate dynamite sex or being an intimate sexual team in dealing with dysfunctional experiences. Affirming first-class female sexuality involves acceptance of the range of sexual roles, meanings, and outcomes.

Summary

A core concept is that female sexuality is first class, not inferior to male sexuality. Female sexuality is variable, flexible, complex, individualistic, and most important, healthy. Women and men function best when they accept each other as intimate and erotic friends. Sexuality is not the most important part of a woman or relationship but has a positive 15–20% role of energizing your bond and reinforcing feelings of desire and desirability. Feeling first class is the opposite of performance anxiety and perfectionism; it's about acceptance and turning toward your partner in good and bad times. First-class sexuality embraces the mantra of desire/pleasure/eroticism/satisfaction. Recognize that desire—especially responsive desire—is the key to sexuality.

When women and men accept the female—male equity model and are intimate and erotic friends, couple sexuality is vibrant and satisfying. You acknowledge the multiple roles, meanings, and outcomes of sexuality. Turn toward your partner in accepting wonderful, good, mediocre, and dissatisfying sexual encounters. GES emphasizes sharing pleasure and accepting the complexity of couple sexuality.

4

INTEGRATING INTIMACY, PLEASURING, AND EROTICISM

Your challenge is to integrate intimacy, nondemand pleasuring, and eroticism in your relationship. In the traditional male—female double standard intimacy was the woman's domain and eroticism the man's. This split subverts female and couple sexuality. In a satisfying sexual relationship both partners value intimacy, pleasuring, and eroticism. Your challenge is to find your "sexual voice," especially your "erotic voice." The challenge for the man is to value intimacy and nondemand pleasuring for himself as well as the relationship.

Healthy sexuality fosters integration and confronts splitting. Reinforce the traditional female focus on emotional and sexual intimacy as well as the value of touch and nondemand pleasuring. You have a right to your sexual voice and to enjoy affectionate, sensual, and playful touch. This isn't just to set the stage for arousal, intercourse, and orgasm; intimacy and nondemand pleasuring are valuable for themselves. He's not giving in or trying to please you. It is his responsibility to value these for himself. When both the woman and man value intimacy/pleasuring/eroticism you experience strong, resilient sexual desire. You are intimate and erotic allies who build a couple sexual style.

Ideally, both partners value intimacy/pleasuring/eroticism. The traditional split by gender has to be confronted; it sets up the male—female power struggle over intercourse. Like all power struggles, it is destructive for the woman, man, and couple. At its essence, sexuality is an intimate team experience, not an adversarial right—wrong conflict. Sadly, traditional gender socialization reinforces the split between intimacy and eroticism, and between women and men (McCarthy & Ross, 2017). The classic power struggle is when the woman says he doesn't care about her intimacy needs; he wants intercourse so he can feel virile. The man counterattacks saying you pretended to love him and want sex, but now you say "no" and avoid being sexual. You demonize each other and fear being the "loser." You are not speaking the same sexual language and are not on the same sexual team.

A strength of the intimacy/pleasuring/eroticism mantra is it gives you a shared language and emphasizes that the couple value each dimension. Intimacy is not only a female characteristic; intimacy belongs to the man and couple. Nondemand pleasuring is the foundation for sexual response. He embraces sharing pleasure as healthier than sex performance. Sharing pleasure is a couple concept in contrast to individual sex performance. You have a right to your sexual voice which includes your erotic voice. Women and men share erotic scenarios and techniques rather than perform for or prove something to the partner.

Intimacy/pleasuring/eroticism is more than its component parts. Integration of these dimensions makes the difference. Intimacy is very different than eroticism, but not incompatible or adversarial. Intimacy is about warm feelings, pleasurable touch, attachment, loving acceptance, security—a predictable, caring relationship. Eroticism is about sexual vitality, taking emotional and sexual risks, not being "socially acceptable," creativity and mystery, intense feelings and sensations, lustful and dramatic scenarios, and unpredictable sexuality. Find your unique integration of intimacy and eroticism so sexual desire is strong and resilient.

Nondemand pleasuring is a crucial dimension, emphasizing the importance of sensual and playful touch. The core of couple sexuality is giving and receiving pleasure-oriented touch rather than sex as an individual performance. Touching is often a bridge to arousal, intercourse, and orgasm. The key for nondemand pleasuring is that sensual and playful touching is valued for itself. Too many couples fall into the traditional male—female power struggle over intercourse. They have only two dimensions of touch-affection and intercourse. If you feel receptive and responsive to touch, the pressure is that it must proceed to intercourse. This results in less touching and less intercourse. Nondemand pleasuring challenges this dichotomy/power struggle by validating the healthy function of sensual and playful touch. On a 10-point scale of subjective arousal, 1–3 sensual pleasure, 4–5 playful touch, 6–9 arousal and erotic flow, and 10 orgasm. Affectionate touch (holding hands, hugging, and kissing) is very important and anchors the couple at 1 in terms of attachment. However, affectionate touch is not sexual. Sensual, playful, and erotic touch as well as intercourse are sexual. You need to confront "sex=intercourse." Sensual, playful, and erotic touch are sexual dimensions. Pleasuring is valuable for itself. This is core in confronting the rigidity of sex=intercourse. Sensual and playful dates are a prime strategy to recognize the value of the variable, flexible couple approach to sexuality. Lesbian couples are particularly comfortable with nondemand pleasuring.

To challenge rigid stereotypes, have the man initiate a sensual date and the woman a playful date. Sensual touch includes back, head, and foot rubs, non-genital body massage, cuddling on the couch listening to music or watching a video, kissing and stroking before going to bed or on awakening. Receptivity and responsivity to touch promotes healthy sexuality.

Playful touch involves genital and non-genital pleasuring and facilitates subjective arousal of 4–5. Playful touch includes whole body massage (with or without a lotion), romantic or erotic dancing, "making out/playing around," touching while showering or bathing, a game like strip poker or Twister. Not all sexuality needs to be intimate or serious. Playful touch is different than sensual or erotic touch. Of course, playful touch can transition to arousal, intercourse, and orgasm, but its core role is sharing pleasure.

Erotic Scenarios and Techniques

Eroticism is the most contentious dimension of the intimacy/pleasuring/eroticism mantra. There is more misunderstanding and bad advice about eroticism than almost any aspect of sexuality. Eroticism based on porn, dramatic sexuality, proving something to yourself or your partner, pressure to act out erotic fantasies, or to be totally free and uninhibited is counter-productive. This intimidates you rather than empowers you. Eroticism is best integrated within the desire/pleasure/eroticism/

satisfaction mantra. Integrated eroticism reinforces your unique "erotic voice."

There are three primary eroticism/arousal styles:

1. Partner interaction arousal focuses on giving and receiving touch. This is the type of sexuality seen in R-rated movies. Each partner's arousal is arousing for the other—the "give to get" pleasure guideline. Partner interaction eroticism/arousal is by far the most common pattern.
2. Self-entrancement arousal focuses on taking turns as giver and receiver. This format was made popular by the sensate focus exercises. The giving partner provides the type of touching she enjoys rather than trying to second guess him. In the receiving role, you take in pleasure and erotic sensations. You are mindful and actively engaged. This is very different than the passivity of "foreplay." As couples age they are more likely to utilize self-entrancement arousal.
3. Role enactment arousal focuses on external stimuli to enhance eroticism. This can involve watching X-rated videos; using sex toys such as paddles, ropes, handcuffs, clips; playing out an erotic fantasy; being sexual in front of a mirror; enacting a BDSM scenario. This type of eroticism is espoused on the internet and in self-help materials. Although erotically charged for some couples, for many it is a sexual "dud" or even anti-erotic. An erotic fantasy is different than a real-life sexual experience. It provides an erotic charge in fantasy, but if acted out can result in awkwardness and self-consciousness. There is nothing more anti-erotic than self-consciousness.

Erotic scenarios and techniques need to be congruent for the couple and facilitate the pleasuring/eroticism process. Feelings and sensations are in the 6–10 subjective arousal range. Many women experience orgasm with erotic sexuality—manual, oral, rubbing, or vibrator stimulation. Other women prefer being orgasmic during intercourse, typically using multiple stimulation (including erotic fantasies). Few women have the same orgasmic pattern as the male—one orgasm during intercourse using only thrusting. If that is your pattern embrace it but realize that it is not the typical orgasmic pattern.

A core concept of integrated eroticism is that it has value in itself. Eroticism usually flows into intercourse, but if that is the demand then eroticism loses its special value.

Valuing Intimacy/Pleasuring/Eroticism

Ideally, both partners value intimacy/pleasuring/eroticism rather than remain stuck with the traditional male—female split and power struggle. This new mantra is more important than its component parts and reinforces female—male sexual equity. The challenge is to develop your unique erotic voice, not in competition to his. Each partner has a right to their feelings and preferences. Each valuing intimacy/pleasuring/eroticism reinforces sexual health. You are not, nor should you be, sexual clones of each other. Recognize that your intimacy/pleasuring/eroticism feelings and preferences are different than his.

Samantha and Jack

Both Samantha and Jack grew up in traditional families with rigid gender expectations about life generally and sexuality specifically. As an adolescent Samantha bitterly resented that her brothers had more freedom than her. Samantha's mother urged her older brothers to use condoms and bought condoms for them. Mother's message to Samantha was to date and enjoy social activities, but to remain "pure." In school, church, and family, abstinence was the approach to sexuality for women. Samantha and her peers read sexuality articles and talked among themselves (but not with adults) about contraception. Samantha was very aware of the negative psychological, medical, and social consequences of sex for adolescent girls. Sadly, there was little discussion of intimacy, nondemand pleasuring, or eroticism.

Samantha's life dramatically changed when she was 16. Her 20-year-old brother got a girlfriend pregnant causing great family drama. They married and separated within the year creating more tension than she'd ever seen between her parents. Samantha's reaction was to become sexually active with a focus on erotic sexuality (but not for positive reasons). Samantha's sexual experiences were not about intimacy and certainly not nondemand pleasuring. She began intercourse at 18 when she and her best friend went to Planned Parenthood for the birth control pill. College dating and sexuality was positive. Samantha was a conscientious birth control user (an IUD—a long acting reversible contraceptive—LARC) and insisted her partner wear a condom to protect against HIV/STI. Although she did occasionally engage in "hook up" sex, she preferred sexual friendships which lasted between a semester and two years. For Samantha, life got better after college and much better after she met Jack at 25.

Samantha was a responsible, independent, "new woman" who wanted a career and a secure relationship, including healthy sexuality. Jack was 24, also a college graduate, who was seeking an equitable emotional and sexual relationship. He was completing his master's degree and planned to teach at a community college. He was not intimidated by Samantha's career and salary (she was a financial analyst). The first year of their relationship celebrated the romantic love/passionate sex/idealization (limerance) phase. This was a wonderful way to begin as a couple. Samantha realized that the limerance phase was time-limited, but that didn't stop her from embracing the special feelings. She realized Jack was more of a romanticist than she which was fine as long as he dealt with the reality of sharing their lives, including developing a couple sexual style after the limerance phase.

Samantha wanted a couple sexual style which integrated intimacy, nondemand pleasuring, and erotic scenarios and techniques. The hardest issue for Jack was nondemand pleasuring. The hardest for Samantha was maintaining her erotic voice—not being overwhelmed by Jack's intercourse focus. Jack got easy, spontaneous erections and wanted to move to intercourse as soon as she was ready. Jack was an engaged lover who was open to Samantha's feelings and preferences, which she appreciated. She didn't want a traditional man who believed he was the master of sex with female sexuality as second class. Samantha saw herself as a healthy sexual woman whose feelings and preferences were as important as his. Jack understood that Samantha valued intimacy/pleasuring/eroticism. She enjoyed intercourse but wanted him to be aware that sexuality was more than intercourse and not all touching had to or should result in intercourse. Especially important was accepting nondemand pleasuring as valuable for itself, not just as a bridge to intercourse.

It takes most couples three—six months to develop a couple sexual style after the limerance phase. With Samantha taking the lead with her pro-sexual approach, this was easily accomplished. An intimate, secure attachment was paramount. Samantha valued that Jack wanted a satisfying, secure bond. They hoped this relationship would lead to marriage. Samantha had seen too many of her girlfriends dramatically fall in love, only later to discover hidden issues which caused a fatally flawed relationship. Samantha and Jack shared their personal, relational, and sexual strengths and vulnerabilities. She wanted to be sure he was "the one" and they could create a satisfying, secure, and sexual marriage.

Implementing nondemand pleasuring was a challenge. Samantha particularly enjoyed giving and receiving back rubs. At times this led to intercourse, but usually it was for sensual pleasure. For Jack, giving a back rub was exciting and a cue for sex. Samantha did not want to feel pushed or be stuck in the role of sexual gatekeeper. This would reduce the sensual pleasure she felt with the back rub.

Nondemand pleasuring is about embracing sensual and playful touch (subjective arousal of 1–5). It is about breaking the traditional male—female power struggle of intercourse or nothing. Pleasuring provides a way to connect and re-connect. Ideally, this results in more touching and more intercourse. Samantha and Jack learned to be comfortable and feel like an intimate team rather than struggle over the role and meaning of pleasuring. Jack did not feel sexually rejected, he realized Samantha truly valued sensual and playful touch. The key for Samantha was freedom to initiate intercourse when she wanted. When she didn't want intercourse, she stayed physically connected rather than turning away.

Developing erotic scenarios and techniques is a challenge. Samantha enjoyed receiving and giving erotic stimulation. Jack preferred giving oral stimulation rather than manual stimulation and enjoyed receiving both oral and manual stimulation. He particularly enjoyed mutual oral stimulation which Samantha found less erotic. She preferred taking turns, although at times would engage in mutual oral pleasuring. They developed an erotic scenario where he gave oral stimulation and received manual stimulation. Samantha preferred mutual stimulation and multiple stimulation. She was open to asynchronous sexual scenarios including pleasuring Jack to orgasm, mixing manual and oral stimulation. She finished with manual stimulation since she did not enjoy his ejaculating in her mouth.

Samantha, like many women, found it easier to be orgasmic with erotic stimulation than with intercourse. For Samantha the key for intercourse was to transition at 7 or 8 subjective arousal and use multiple stimulation during intercourse. This included giving and receiving stimulation, especially manual clitoral stimulation, receiving buttock stimulation, giving testicle stimulation, and freedom to use private erotic fantasies as a bridge to erotic flow.

A key issue was Jack's desire to switch to intercourse quickly. Samantha was open to this when she was not desirous of being orgasmic. Samantha did not need to be orgasmic each time nor need orgasm in order to feel satisfied. She experienced orgasm in over 80% of encounters whether with oral stimulation before intercourse, during intercourse using multiple stimulation, or with manual stimulation during afterplay. A preferred scenario was Samantha being orgasmic with oral stimulation before intercourse, multiple stimulation during intercourse, and multiple orgasms in afterplay (Kleimplatz & Menard, 2007). Jack joked that she had ten times more pleasure than he, but that was not Samantha's experience. She liked that erotic sex had different roles, meanings, and outcomes. Jack was her intimate and erotic ally. They built desire/pleasure/eroticism/satisfaction patterns which would continue throughout their life.

Maintaining Intimacy/Pleasuring/Eroticism

It is easier to develop than to maintain intimacy/pleasuring/eroticism. With the reality of jobs, children, household responsibilities, community activities, sexuality can slip into a lesser role. A common pattern is that couples fall into a routine so even if sex is functional it is not special or energizing. Don't let sexuality rest on its laurels or fall into a mechanical pattern. You owe it to yourself and your relationship to value intimacy/pleasuring/eroticism. Men tolerate mediocre/marginal sex easier than women. If sex falls into a mediocre pattern, you have a high risk of developing low sexual desire. You want sex worth having.

Valuing intimacy/pleasuring/eroticism prevents falling into the trap of a marginal sexual relationship. Nondemand pleasuring facilitates a variable, flexible approach to sensual and playful touch. This confronts routine, mechanical sex. Cuddling and playful touch is a bridge to sexual desire as well as a means to share pleasure. Erotic scenarios and techniques invite sexual experimentation and create special turn-ons. The core function of eroticism is to promote sexual vitality. Routine, predictable sex (even if functional) does not energize you or your bond. Erotic play and experimentation is special and enhances strong, resilient desire.

Intimacy/pleasuring/eroticism is more than its component parts. The integration of these three dimensions provides strong, resilient sexual desire and facilitates genuine, satisfying couple sexuality.

Exercise: Creating Intimacy/Pleasuring/Eroticism

This exercise makes personal and concrete the mantra of intimacy/pleasuring/eroticism. You take the first initiation. Each person's scenario will be different; you are not clones of each other. Be sure your scenario integrates all three dimensions.

Create a unique scenario where the whole is more than each component. Initiate in a manner which promotes the level of intimacy which invites a sexual encounter. Too much intimacy smothers sexual risk-taking and results in de-eroticizing your partner. Too little intimacy results in a sex performance to prove something to the partner. Find the balance of intimacy that facilitates warmth and attachment while inviting eroticism and risk-taking.

You can begin the encounter standing, sitting, or laying down; in the living room, on the deck, or in the bedroom; dressed, semi-dressed, or nude; starting with affectionate, sensual, or playful touch; verbal or non-verbal; serious or silly. What allows you to feel intimately connected and facilitates sexual desire? How can he help set the sexual mood?

What is your preferred way to share nondemand pleasuring? Do you intermix affectionate, sensual, and playful touch? Do you prefer giving and receiving at the same time (partner interaction arousal) or taking turns (self-entrancement arousal)? Does talking facilitate pleasure or do you prefer to let your fingers do the talking? Does using a lotion facilitate pleasurable sensations? Do you enjoy cuddling, stroking, scratching, massage, playful touch? Do you enjoy mixing non-genital and genital touch or does a single focus promote pleasure?

How do you make the transition from pleasuring to eroticism? Do you mix pleasurable and sexual touch, or do you focus on erotic feelings and sensations? Do you prefer manual, oral, or rubbing stimulation? Do you value erotic play or do you want to quickly proceed to orgasm? Do you enjoy a mutual synchronous experience or is asynchronous eroticism a better fit for you? Don't try to second guess your partner or be "politically correct." Go with your erotic feelings and preferences. Give yourself permission to enjoy intense sensations and feelings. Enjoy integrated intimacy/pleasuring/eroticism.

At a different time, he has an opportunity to create and play out his intimacy/pleasuring/eroticism scenario. This is not a competition nor are you clones. Enjoy his unique scenario.

> Remember, the focus of this exercise is both partners valuing intimacy/pleasuring/eroticism. The whole is more than the parts.

Confronting Gender Stereotypes

Traditionally, women and men received very different sexual socialization. Women valued intimacy and nondemand pleasuring and men valued eroticism (especially intercourse and orgasm). It is easy to say that women and men can learn to value intimacy/pleasuring/eroticism, but implementing this new mantra is a challenge. Integrated eroticism leads to enhanced sexual function and satisfaction for the woman and couple.

A key is to change attitudes, behavior, and feelings in a congruent manner. Sexuality is an emotional/behavioral experience, not just cognitions and expectations. Be honest with yourself and your partner. Attitudinally, behaviorally, and emotionally accept the intimacy/pleasuring/eroticism mantra. If there is a dimension which is difficult for you or you feel ambivalent about, share this concern with your partner. Silence and embarrassment gives the problem more power which makes the situation worse. For example, contrary to gender stereotypes, many women have difficulty with intimacy or nondemand pleasuring. Perhaps you felt manipulated or misused rather than accepted and supported in your relationship history. You might feel uncomfortable with the vulnerability of intimacy. Or you feel good about emotional intimacy, but anxious with sexual intimacy. Rather than being silent or feeling guilty, turn toward your partner and share your concerns and feelings. The change process is a combination of personal responsibility and being an intimate sexual team. He is your partner in building comfort and confidence with sexual intimacy, nondemand pleasuring, and erotic scenarios. However, he can't do it for you. Reinforcing the value of your intimate sexual bond is crucial to the change process. Intimacy involves both positive feelings and dealing with problems. No person or relationship is perfect. Intimacy is about feeling close, loved, and accepted with your strengths and vulnerabilities.

A key to sexual intimacy is feeling receptive and responsive to affectionate, sensual, and playful touch.

Some women feel uncomfortable and uncertain about nondemand pleasuring. Her experience is that once sensual or playful touching begins (and he has an erection) it has to lead to intercourse. Be aware of your authentic feelings and choices. Freedom, choice, and unpredictability enhance sexual desire. You have a right to enjoy nondemand pleasuring. His erection is a sign he is experiencing pleasure rather than a demand for intercourse and orgasm. Sensual and playful dates with a prohibition on intercourse and orgasm is an impactful way to make the concept of nondemand pleasuring personal and concrete.

A key to acceptance of eroticism is its integration into the intimacy/pleasuring/eroticism mantra rather than eroticism as an individual performance to prove something to the partner or self. Integrated eroticism is core for healthy female and couple sexuality. Eroticism belongs to you and your relationship. You have a right to choose partner interaction arousal, self-entrancement arousal, role enactment arousal, or a combination of these. You have the right to veto erotic scenarios and techniques that do not fit your feelings and preferences. Embrace your "erotic voice" including your "orgasmic voice."

Summary

A key concept is that the intimacy/pleasuring/eroticism mantra is more than its component parts. This is motivating and empowering for the woman and couple. You have the power to confront and change attitudes, behaviors, and feelings which subvert intimacy/pleasuring/eroticism. It is your responsibility to institute these changes and turn toward your partner as your intimate and your erotic ally. You deserve to enjoy sexuality as a first-class woman and couple. An integral component of healthy female and couple sexuality is embracing awareness that sexuality is more than intercourse. Intimacy promotes a close, secure bond; nondemand pleasuring promotes sensual and playful feelings;

and eroticism promotes intense sensations and feelings which include intercourse and orgasm.

The woman, man, couple, and culture embracing intimacy/pleasuring/eroticism promotes sexual desire and satisfaction. Intimacy, pleasuring, and eroticism are different dimensions, but can be integrated and the whole is more than the parts.

5

DESIRE: THE CORE OF SEXUALITY

Traditionally, professionals and the public believed that male sexuality was superior to female sexuality. The male model of spontaneous erection, erotic fantasy, intercourse, and orgasm was the "natural" path for sexual desire. Whether explained by biological factors (testosterone), gender factors (masculinity), or social factors (men value sexuality more than women), the assumption was that male desire was natural and superior.

There is an overwhelming body of scientific and clinical evidence which challenges these assumptions. The new scientific concept is that female sexual desire is first class, not inferior. Female desire is more complex, variable, flexible, individualistic, and, most important, healthy. Female and male sexuality are different (especially in adolescence and young adulthood), but not adversarial or incompatible. This is not a competition, but an understanding that women and men function best when they are intimate and erotic friends.

As mentioned previously, a little known scientific reality is that when couples become non-sexual it is almost always the man's choice, made unilaterally and conveyed non-verbally. He has lost confidence in erections, intercourse, and orgasm. Males learn sexual desire and response as easy, predictable, and autonomous (he needs nothing from the woman to experience desire, erection, and ejaculation). Most women learn sexuality as intimate, interactive, variable, and flexible. In the long term, the female model of desire and function promotes healthy sexuality, especially in a married or partnered relationship and with aging.

The breakthrough concept is "responsive female sexual desire" rather than spontaneous, autonomous desire (Basson, 2001). You engage in giving and receiving touch and are open to your emotions and those of your partner. You often begin the encounter at neutral, but when you are receptive and responsive to touching and sensual feelings, this is when you experience desire. Desire is responsive to touch and emotions rather than spontaneous and orgasm-driven. Instead of traditional "foreplay" where he stimulated you with the goal of being ready for intercourse, nondemand pleasuring involves giving and receiving sensual and playful touch. A crucial difference is that you are actively involved rather than passive. Sensual and playful touch is valued for itself as well as the potential (not demand) to transition to intercourse.

The new sexual mantra is desire/pleasure/eroticism/satisfaction. Desire is the most important dimension. The key to desire is anticipation of pleasure. Rather than the traditional male—female power struggle of intercourse or nothing, accept sensual, playful, and erotic touch as integral to couple sexuality. It is crucial to confront the "sex=intercourse" myth. Intercourse is integral to the pleasuring/eroticism process, but sexuality is much more than intercourse. When intercourse is viewed as a pass–fail sex test this increases performance anxiety which decreases sexual desire. Responsive female desire is based on choice and a broad-based understanding of the roles, meanings, and outcomes of sexuality (Brotto & Luria, 2014). This approach to desire is healthy for the woman, man, couple, and culture. This focus on pleasure is in sharp contrast to the adolescent and young adult experiences of being pressured sexually, especially sexual harassment and sexual assault.

Desire is facilitated by the cognition that you deserve sexual pleasure. Your sense of deserving is not contingent on everything being perfect—body image, relationship, family, household. Pleasure is your right as a woman. Freedom, choice, playfulness, and unpredictability promote desire.

Sexual desire is subverted by anticipatory and performance anxiety, anger and coercion, alienation, and routine, totally predictable sex.

Physiologically, anything which is good for your body is good for your sexuality. Physical health, including healthy behavioral habits of sleep, exercise, and eating promotes sexual desire and function. It is not aging, but illness and side-effects of medications which subvert sexual function. Fears and distress about the medical problem alter sexual function. The key to maintaining sexual desire with illness and disability is to focus on anticipation and deserving sexual pleasure, not feel controlled by sex performance fears. Sexually, you accept the "new normal." Illness, disability, and the side-effects of medications alter sexual function, but do not stop sexuality, especially not sexual desire.

Relationship factors are crucial for sexual desire. Contrary to public and media assumptions, communication and intimacy is not the answer for desire problems. The key is viewing your spouse (partner) as both an intimate and erotic friend. Intimacy and eroticism are different dimensions, but not adversarial or incompatible. A key challenge is to value your "erotic voice." Eroticism is an integral component of healthy female and couple sexuality. Integrate intimacy and eroticism into your relationship. So many women say, "I love my spouse, but am not in love with him." They have de-eroticized the spouse and relationship. Intimacy is about warm, loving, close, secure feelings of attachment. Eroticism is about taking emotional and sexual risks, creativity, mystery, intense sensations and feelings, and unpredictability. Both are necessary for sexual desire and healthy sexuality.

In creating your couple sexual style, the issue is your "sexual voice" (autonomy) balanced with being an intimate team who integrates intimacy and eroticism. Your sexual voice includes your "erotic voice." The traditional gender split had the woman valuing intimacy and security while the man valued eroticism and intercourse. The assumption was that men and women were very different sexually. The sexual equity model is based on acceptance of healthy female desire and function. Both partners value desire/pleasure/eroticism/satisfaction. In married/partnered relationships, sexual similarities far outweigh differences. The key is acceptance and openness to change. Your challenge is to value sexuality generally and eroticism specifically. Do not reduce the value of intimacy and security, rather enhance and broaden it to value eroticism, orgasm, intercourse, and the energizing role of sexuality for yourself and your relationship.

The challenge for the man is to value intimacy, a broad approach to sexual pleasure, and the importance of relational meaning and security. Sex is not an individual performance with a pass–fail intercourse test. Sexuality is about sharing pleasure and valuing sensual, playful, and erotic touch in addition to intercourse. This does not diminish intercourse or orgasm. It enhances variable, flexible, broad-based sexuality and sex as a team sport.

Pleasuring vs. Foreplay

One in three adult women reports low or inhibited sexual desire. That is a sad and depressing statistic. The clinical term is Female Sexual Interest/Arousal Disorder (FSIAD). Like other sexual problems desire issues are multi-causal, multi-dimensional with large individual, couple, cultural, and value differences. Psychological, bio-medical, and social/relational factors need to be carefully assessed and understood (Brotto & Woo, 2010). Common psychological causes are not valuing sexuality, history of sexual trauma, negative emotions (anger, anxiety, depression), poor body image, and not having a positive sexual voice. Bio-medical factors include sexual pain, fear of pregnancy or sexually transmitted infections, illness and side-effects of medications, alcohol or drug abuse, and poor behavioral health habits. Social/relational factors include de-eroticizing the partner, power struggles over intercourse frequency, sexual demands or coercion, focus on foreplay rather than pleasuring, conflict over erotic techniques, avoidance because of a sex dysfunction (whether his or hers) and sexual putdowns. Sexual desire is very easy to kill.

A common factor negating female desire is the scenario where the man initiates sex with the focus on "foreplay" to get you ready for intercourse. All sensual and sexual touch results in intercourse. If you insist on "no," this results in an argument or the traditional power struggle where he puts you down as non-sexual and you counter-attack saying he is sexually selfish. Power struggles are unhealthy for the woman, man, and couple. The issue is not being the "loser"—if you have intercourse you lose, if no intercourse he is the loser. In this struggle, it is hard to see the role of first-class female and couple sexual desire.

The solution is to confront the "intercourse or nothing" power struggle. Traditional "foreplay" needs to be eliminated because it raises self-consciousness and performance anxiety while lowering anticipation and pleasure. The foreplay scenario is replaced by both partners valuing sensual touch, playful touch, erotic touch, as well as intercourse. You are sexually aware and active, not passive. Valuing nondemand pleasuring is especially important.

This allows you to have your voice, to enjoy giving and receiving pleasure without the demand aspect of "foreplay." Embrace eroticism as an integral component of your sexual voice. Eroticism is integrated into the desire/pleasure/eroticism/satisfaction mantra. Rather than feeling intimidated or turned-off by the porn model of eroticism, embrace eroticism as a sexual woman who desires vibrant, satisfying sexuality. Whether emphasizing partner interaction, self-entrancement, or role enactment arousal scenarios, you experience high levels of sexual intensity, creativity, mystery, take personal and sexual risks, enjoy unpredictable scenarios, and vibrant sexuality as your sexual right. Choose whether to incorporate role enactment arousal scenarios to provide an erotic charge for you, not to perform for or prove anything to your partner. Do not allow yourself to be intimidated by comparisons with porn videos; accept your unique erotic preferences. Allow eroticism to enhance your sexual voice and desire.

Sexual satisfaction is facilitated by acceptance and positive, realistic expectations. Most important is the Good Enough Sex (GES) model. GES values variable, flexible couple sexuality rather than demanding perfect individual sex performance. The best example involves orgasm. Rather than following the male model of one predictable orgasm during intercourse, healthy female sexuality emphasizes accepting your unique orgasmic pattern. This is true whether your pattern involves orgasm during erotic stimulation (before or after intercourse), orgasm during intercourse using multiple stimulation (with a special focus on clitoral stimulation and erotic fantasy), multi-orgasmic response during cunnilingus, rubbing stimulation to orgasm, experiencing an emission during orgasm, a "G-spot" orgasm, or your unique orgasmic pattern. Many women experience orgasm with two or more scenarios. What is the percent of time you are orgasmic during couple sex? Few women are orgasmic 95–100% of experiences, although if that is your pattern own it. The average orgasmic response during couple sex is 70% of experiences—the range is 30–90%. Rather than "one right way to be orgasmic," the healthy approach is to own and accept your orgasmic pattern. Sexual satisfaction is enhanced by acceptance and subverted by performance demands.

Desire is facilitated by positive, realistic sexual expectations. The healthy cycle is pleasure-oriented sex and a regular rhythm of sexuality which emphasizes multiple roles, meanings, and GES outcomes.

Bio-Medical Interventions

The drug companies, spurred by profits from the pro-erection medications, hope to market medications to enhance female sexual desire. Addyi was the first medication to receive FDA approval in 2015. We advocate for the comprehensive psychobiosocial approach for the assessment and treatment of female (and male) sexual problems, but warn against use of a medication as a stand-alone intervention. This is particularly relevant for Addyi which is a relatively weak medication with limited therapeutic impact (McCarthy, Koman, & Cohn, 2018).

When the woman lacks any testosterone, using testosterone enhancement via a patch or gel form can be a valuable bio-medical intervention to enhance desire. However, like Addyi, it will not be effective as a stand-alone intervention. Many women are motivated by the concept that to enhance desire you need three integrated resources. Finding your sexual voice serves a one-third role; Addyi or testosterone enhancement can build sexual anticipation and enthusiasm which provides a one-third resource; and enlisting your partner as your intimate and erotic ally provides the most important one-third. This psychobiosocial approach to build sexual desire is likely to be effective. Hopefully, in the future there will be better bio-medical resources which are more efficacious and user-friendly. However, you can't ask a drug to do it all. You deserve a positive sexual voice and a couple sexual style that integrates intimacy, pleasuring, and eroticism to promote strong, resilient sexual desire.

Bridges to Sexual Desire

An empowering, motivating strategy is "bridges to sexual desire." Rather than hoping for spontaneous and easy sex, accept that the majority of sexual encounters are planned or semi-planned. This is especially true for women who work, have children, and community responsibilities. It is important to have your bridges to desire rather than ceding sexual initiation to your partner.

A core factor is that unless you have the power to say "no" to sex, you don't have the freedom to say "yes" to sex. The right to veto a sexual scenario or technique is crucial for first-class female sexuality. You trust he will honor your veto. Veto does not mean sexual avoidance. Turn toward your partner and initiate a sensual, playful, erotic, or intercourse experience. Avoidance feeds on itself and sex becomes the enemy. Intimacy, pleasuring, and eroticism are integral to desire.

In R-rated movies, the woman is turned-on before any touching occurs. For the majority of adult women, pleasure-oriented touch is the key to sexual desire. When you are open to giving and receiving nondemand pleasuring, sexual receptivity and responsivity increase. Ideally, you are open to "her," "his," and "our" bridges to desire. Contrary to romantic love myths, it is unusual for both partners to have the same preferences for sexual initiation. You are not sexual clones. It is normal and healthy to have different ways to initiate sex. Positive anticipation is the key to sexual desire. Invite him to join you sexually. Be open to his initiation/bridges and together create "our" bridges to desire.

Exercise: Developing Your Bridges to Sexual Desire

Desire is an example of the adage, "Sexually one size never fits all." This exercise asks you to develop your unique bridges to desire.

Begin with the milieu. Would you like to start in the bedroom, in front of the fireplace, sitting on the deck with a glass of wine, take a walk and engage in playful touching? Is your initiation verbal or non-verbal? Do you want to begin with sensual touch or have a quick warm-up and move to intercourse? What is most sexually inviting: partner interaction arousal, self-entrancement arousal, or role enactment arousal? Is your preference to be orgasmic with manual, oral, rubbing, intercourse, or vibrator stimulation? Do you prefer multiple stimulation or one focused stimulation? Afterplay is the most ignored component of sexuality—what is your favorite afterplay scenario?

The core of desire is personally inviting sexual scenario(s). Don't be passive, expect the man to be the expert, or let him take the sexual lead. Your sexual voice and preferences are as important as his. It's okay if preferences and bridges are different. Maintaining desire is a couple challenge and facilitates variable, flexible sexuality rather than routine, predictable sex. Your bridges reinforce anticipation, deserving, choice, and freedom. A key for strong, resilient desire is to value your unique sexual voice. This does not negate his sexual voice—it is complementary, facilitating vital and satisfying couple sexuality.

Danielle and Stuart

Danielle was 38 years old, married for nine years to 37-year-old Stuart. Danielle had a 14-year-old son from a previous relationship. Stuart legally adopted the son and they were hoping to conceive a baby. Intercourse with the goal of pregnancy was a sexual aphrodisiac for Danielle.

Danielle felt better about herself as a sexual woman than any time in her life. Her body image and sexual self-esteem had never been higher. She felt like a first-class woman.

Her mother died when Danielle was 9, her father quickly remarried, and even more quickly divorced. He had several girlfriends, remarrying again when Danielle was 14 to a woman who was critical of Danielle's clothes, activities, and quite concerned about sexuality, especially fearful of Danielle becoming pregnant. As an adolescent, friends told her she was attractive, but Danielle didn't feel attractive. At 16 Danielle asked her step-mother to accompany her to Planned Parenthood to obtain birth control pills, but she refused. Danielle hated the pressure of the dating/sex games in high school. She occasionally had intercourse using condoms, but preferred manual sex which entailed no risk of pregnancy. She felt intimidated by how easily the adolescent male obtained an erection while her arousal lagged behind.

When Danielle entered college, her view of life and sexuality greatly improved. Danielle was proud that she was the first in her family to graduate college; she was a "new woman"—a perspective reinforced by her peer group. This included being a conscientious birth control user whether she was involved in a serious relationship or not. She knew too many friends who had unwanted pregnancies, some of whom had abortions and others became single mothers.

Danielle preferred having a steady boyfriend (a "sexual friend"). Those relationships lasted 6–18 months. She was not averse to "hook-up" sex which was exciting and unpredictable but stayed away from "players." In her junior year, Danielle took a human sexuality class where she earned an "A." Most important, she learned psychological, biological, and relational information. Danielle felt empowered by that class to be a first-class sexual woman. She illustrated the adage "Knowledge is power."

Danielle's post-college life involved a significant split between professional success and relational/sexual problems. Danielle was accepted into a corporate training program where she thrived and received two promotions. Unfortunately, she became involved in a romantic love/passionate sex affair with a 42-year-old vice-president. The relationship was dramatic and sexually driven. He told Danielle he had a vasectomy so she need not use birth control. Danielle was hesitant, but he lobbied hard insisting this demonstrated her commitment to him. He promised he would leave his wife and have the vasectomy reversed. Danielle felt swept away with the promise of this relationship. She felt sexually free, not burdened by birth control. Four months later, her optimism and enthusiasm for the relationship had waned. She learned he had been passed over for promotion and was not respected in the organization. She heard rumors of past affairs with young trainees. The "straw that broke the camel's back" was meeting his wife and three of their four children at a firm picnic.

Shortly afterward, Danielle discovered she was pregnant. At first, he was angry and blamed her for having sex with another man. Danielle insisted on a paternity test, confirming that he was the father. After a very painful, humiliating interaction with his lawyer, Danielle accepted a one-time payment of $245,000 for care of the child, with the understanding he would not have contact with Danielle or the baby. In a further destructive move, he tried to have her fired. Danielle used the human resources department and her boss to support her job and right to maternity leave.

Danielle was committed to being a successful professional and single mother. She hired a nanny and mobilized friends and extended family to help. Even though she was not in a relationship, she chose to have an IUD inserted. She planned to resume dating and being sexual. Danielle saw herself as a proud, resilient woman who valued touching and sexuality. If a new man could not accept her life situation, this was his problem, not hers.

Danielle met Stuart when she was 26 and married at 28. During dating and cohabitating ten months before the marriage, Danielle and Stuart carefully discussed each other's psychological, relational, and sexual histories. There are no perfect people and no perfect relationships. Danielle wanted Stuart to know her strengths and vulnerabilities, and she wanted to know his. Sexual attraction was a strength. Danielle enjoyed the romantic love/passionate sex phase. She wanted to be sure that she and Stuart could transition to a couple sexual style of intimacy, pleasuring, and eroticism so that desire remained strong and resilient. Danielle realized sexuality was not a core factor in marital choice, but desired sexuality to have a 15–20% energizing role. She wanted to feel desire and desirable throughout the marriage.

Danielle understood that the first two years of the marriage would be hard work. Practically and emotionally they joined their lives. Stuart legally adopted Danielle's son two years later. Sexuality served as a resource to energize their relationship and keep them motivated to resolve difficult issues. Danielle accepted the positive function of "quickies," especially as a tension reducer for Stuart. She wanted to be sure this was balanced with intimate sexual encounters which met her emotional and sexual needs. Danielle recognized that couple sexuality was variable and flexible. It could play different roles, carry different meanings, and result in different outcomes. The best sex was mutual and synchronous—both Danielle and Stuart experienced desire/pleasure/eroticism/satisfaction. Danielle also valued asynchronous sexuality—sometimes better for Stuart, sometimes better for her. Sex as a refuge or tension reducer was embraced by Danielle; this type of sex is not just for the man.

The decision to have a second child was well thought out. Stuart very much wanted the experience of parenting a baby. Unlike Danielle's first pregnancy, this would be a planned, wanted child with two involved parents. A child is a major life commitment—Danielle was aware she would be almost 60 when this child was launched to college. Having a baby with Stuart, cooperative parenting, and experiencing the child's development was a strong motivator. Sex with the intention of pregnancy was an aphrodisiac. They conceived in their third month which was a joy as well as a relief from the fear of fertility problems at her age. Danielle wanted to stay sexual throughout the pregnancy, including the last trimester. She especially enjoyed intercourse in the sitting position with Stuart kneeling in front of her. There was no pressure on her stomach/uterus. This is a wonderful position for multiple stimulation. When intercourse was not desired, they remained physically connected with sensual, playful, and erotic scenarios.

Danielle and Stuart attended prepared childbirth classes. The delivery was enhanced by his support and her using breathing, relaxation, and mindfulness techniques. The birth was a special day in her life.

Danielle and Stuart vowed to be in the 30% of couples who maintain vital couple sexuality while parenting. Touching and sexuality energized their bond. Danielle wanted to feel desire and desirable as a wife, not just a mother. With less time, energy, and space to be sexual, desire would still remain a personal and couple priority. Most of their sexual encounters were planned or semi-planned, with the necessity of working around the children's schedules. Danielle had thought sexuality was most challenging in the baby phase, but was surprised that the biggest challenge in terms of time and planning was when children are adolescents. Danielle and Stuart planned a couple weekend away without children at least once a year. The logistics of babysitting with a back-up system in case of emergency was not easy, but very worthwhile.

Couple friends experienced a major drama when the woman had an intense affair with someone from work. Affairs are an example of sexual behavior being multi-causal, multi-dimensional, with large individual, couple, cultural, and value differences. Like most affairs, the marriage survived, but with much turmoil and distress. Danielle did not want that type of disruption in her life and family. Danielle and Stuart were in careers and work travel which provided opportunity for affairs. Their primary prevention strategy included frank discussions and an emotional/behavioral agreement to reinforce their monogamy commitment. First, they identified and disclosed what type of mood, person, and situation would make each spouse vulnerable to an affair. Danielle had assumed they would have similar vulnerabilities and was quite surprised to learn that Stuart's vulnerabilities were very different than hers. For Danielle, the vulnerable mood was depression, the situation was feeling alone and disconnected, and the potential partner would be an emotionally needy man. Danielle made an emotional commitment to tell Stuart if she was in a vulnerable situation and discuss this before acting on the impulse (Stuart agreed to this for himself). They would explore an affair as a decision in the same way they discussed changing jobs, houses, or the child's school. They would process the meaning of a potential affair for the involved spouse, injured spouse, and its role and meaning for the marriage. It would not be an impulsive, secret activity. Third, if there was a physical, emotional, or on-line incident it would be disclosed within 72 hours. The cover-up is more impactful than the affair itself. This agreement allowed Danielle to embrace couple sexuality rather than be afraid that she would impulsively be swept away by an affair or need to be vigilant about Stuart having an affair.

Danielle realized that she could not treat sexuality with "benign neglect." For sex to remain vibrant and satisfying, both she and Stuart needed to be open to new scenarios and techniques. They agreed that at least once a year each spouse would initiate something new—a different pleasuring position or lotion, a surprise initiation, a new afterplay scenario, a different intercourse position or thrusting motion, a sex game or toy, or a different multiple stimulation sequence before or during intercourse. Creative, satisfying sexuality requires new inputs and energy.

Danielle values her sexual voice and is committed to sexuality having a 15–20% role in her life in the present and future.

Embracing Female Sexual Desire

Responsive sexual desire is optimal for the woman and couple. With the aging of the man and relationship he needs your sexual voice to promote male and couple sexuality. Your receptivity and responsivity to touch enhances his sexuality and allows you to be a vital, satisfied couple. He learns to "piggyback" his arousal on yours.

The concept of sexuality as an intimate team sport is true throughout life, even more so with aging. Female sexual desire and responsivity is healthy for you, him, and your relationship. In fact, for many men in their 50s and almost all men in their 60s and older, "responsive male desire" becomes a crucial resource. Rather than depending on spontaneous erection as the cue to desire, both the woman and man are responsive to touch and emotional connection. Desire is enhanced by engagement. Embracing male responsive desire and GES is critical for healthy sexuality in your 60s, 70s, and 80s.

Valuing your sexual voice and enjoying broad-based sexuality—sensual, playful, erotic, and intercourse—is the foundation for sexual desire. Not only is female desire first class, it forms the basis for sexual satisfaction. Recognizing the multiple roles, meanings, and outcomes of sexuality facilitates accepting both synchronous and asynchronous sexual experiences. Rather than sex always having to be warm, loving, and intimate, this approach affirms sex as a tension reducer, sex as a refuge, sex as playful, erotic sex, mundane sex to get through a boring patch, sex as a means for healing, and sex to enhance attachment. Strong, resilient desire is vital for you and your relationship.

Summary

Sexual desire is the core dimension for healthy female and couple sexuality. The breakthrough concept is "responsive female sexual desire." Confront the traditional "common sense" belief that male desire defined by spontaneous erection, autonomous sexual response, and intercourse performance is the definition of "normal" desire. Female sexual desire is variable, flexible, complex, and individualistic. The most important understanding is that female desire is first class. Desire is a response to emotional connection and giving and receiving pleasure-oriented touch. Female desire emphasizes intimate, interactive sexuality including accepting a range of roles, meanings, and outcomes. Female desire values both synchronous and asynchronous sexual experiences. Positive anticipation, sense of deserving pleasure, freedom, choice, and unpredictable scenarios increase desire. Value both intimacy and eroticism and turn toward your partner as your sexual ally. Maintain strong, resilient sexual desire.

6

NONDEMAND PLEASURING

Nondemand pleasuring is the foundation for sexual function. Pleasuring is an integral component of the desire/pleasure/eroticism/satisfaction mantra. The essence of couple sexuality is giving and receiving pleasure-oriented touch. Pleasuring is a couple concept, the antithesis of the individual pass–fail performance model of sex.

Nondemand pleasuring involves both sensual and playful touch. In terms of subjective arousal, pleasuring involves sensations and feelings in the 1–5 range. The roots of nondemand pleasuring are the classic sensate focus exercises (Masters & Johnson, 1970). Sensate focus is the therapeutic technique most employed by couple therapists to deal with sexual problems. Unfortunately, the misguided emphasis has been on the giving partner pleasuring the receiving partner to increase her sexual responsiveness (Weiner & Avery-Clark, 2017). This approach is similar to traditional "foreplay." The therapeutic model of nondemand pleasuring is that the giving partner's focus is on touching for himself—providing a range of pleasurable sensations so you are able to define for yourself pleasurable sensations and feelings. You are actively involved and aware throughout the pleasuring process; not passive as in foreplay. The partner is your sexual friend who presents you with a range of pleasurable touch and sensations. When you are the giving partner, you provide touching you enjoy giving rather than trying to second guess him.

There are two dimensions of nondemand pleasure. First, sensual touch (non-genital) involving subjective arousal in the 1–3 range. Second, playful touch which mixes non-genital and genital pleasuring with subjective arousal range of 4–5. Nondemand pleasuring is a major source for sexual desire and can serve as a bridge to arousal and orgasm. Remember, its chief function is giving and receiving pleasure-oriented touching which is integral to couple sexuality.

The key is the nondemand aspect of touching. Rather than a focus on arousal and performance, nondemand pleasuring focuses on being present, mindful, sharing good feelings/sensations, and experiencing attachment. Pleasure is integral to the sexuality experience. This confronts the traditional "sex=intercourse" myth. Sensual and playful touch serves as the foundation for broad-based, variable, flexible couple sexuality. Nondemand pleasuring is a sexual dimension which is valued for itself. Its secondary function is as a bridge to arousal, intercourse, and orgasm.

Implementing Nondemand Pleasuring

To ensure that nondemand pleasuring is more than a "politically correct" concept, your partner makes a cognitive-behavioral-emotional commitment to integrate pleasuring into the reality of your day-to-day sexual relationship. Many (if not most) couples only have two gears (dimensions) of touch-affection and intercourse. The best way to implement nondemand pleasuring is to schedule at least two, and preferably three, sensual touching dates and follow that with two to three playful touching dates. Usually we do not suggest a prohibition on intercourse, but at this phase of implementing nondemand pleasuring the temporary prohibition is valuable.

Your partner values pleasuring; he does not view it as your domain or as something he does for your sake. Take turns initiating a nondemand pleasuring scenario. When it's your turn play it out in a manner which is special for you. Enjoy the experience outside your bedroom (as long as you have privacy). It could be in the den, living room, guest bedroom, or on the deck late at night. It's your choice whether to do this nude, semi-clothed, or in a sexy outfit. Feel comfortable with the milieu-welcome sharing pleasure.

Common enhancements are a sensual lotion, music in the background, and/or a glass of wine. Do you prefer standing up, lying down, dancing? Do you want to initiate, have him initiate, be seductive or playful, verbal or non-verbal? Is pleasuring more inviting if there is mutual give and take touching (partner interaction arousal) or taking turns with the giver-receiver format (self-entrancement arousal)? Don't try to second guess or please your partner; create a scenario that is inviting for you. When it is his turn, be open to his requests, preferences, and scenarios.

A major challenge is to identify and embrace sensuality, involving subjective sensations and feelings in the 1–3 range. Give yourself permission to be receptive and responsive to sensual touch. Many women find it easier and "natural" to be the giver. In addition, you deserve sensual pleasure—be open to the warm, rhythmic sensations of receiving a non-genital body massage, having your back scratched or your thighs stroked, feeling enveloped in a hug, being kissed and your face caressed. Allow your body to relax. Be mindful of feelings of warmth and comfort. Are you responsive to long, slow, rhythmic touching in contrast to goal-oriented foreplay? As you practice nondemand pleasuring your body becomes attuned to the pleasures of sensuality. Incorporate pleasuring into your couple sexual repertoire.

The next step is to integrate playful touching. Many women and couples find this challenging, but quite valuable. Playful touch integrates genital and non-genital touching. This often involves him getting an erection (or you not overreacting if he does not get an erection). Traditionally, his erection was a cue for intercourse. Rather than welcoming his erection, it felt like performance pressure for intercourse or at least bringing him to orgasm. Women fear being labeled a "sex tease" or his anger driven by sexual frustration. This model of sex is not healthy for the woman, man, couple, or culture. Playful pleasuring introduces new understandings and experiences. Both partners value the 4–5 level of subjective feelings/sensations. It is a different level of pleasure than sensual touch. The challenge is to remain intimate sexual friends. The fact that playful touch elicits an erection is a sign of heightened pleasure, not a demand for intercourse (or orgasm). Enjoy his erection rather than feel intimidated by it. In the same way, welcome your 4–5 level of subjective arousal (which often includes vaginal lubrication and breast swelling). Remind yourself and each other to enjoy sharing pleasure without performance pressure. Playful touch challenges the "common sense" belief that if sex play results in arousal then it should lead to intercourse. For some couples the transition to intercourse occurs 90% of the time, but for most it occurs 70%, 50%, or 20% of the time. Remember, playful touch is a sexual dimension that has value in itself. Without that understanding, you lose freedom and choice which is core to sexual desire. Totally predictable sex where all sensual and playful touch leads to intercourse ultimately reduces desire. Variable, flexible couple sexuality promotes desire and satisfaction (McCarthy & McCarthy, 2014).

In what ways is your playful scenario different than your sensual scenario? Some women find it similar and others have a different way to initiate and enjoy playful touching. For example, some couples prefer the bedroom for a playful scenario while others prefer playing in the living room. Some enjoy a game like strip poker or Twister while others choose to bask in subjective arousal. Whole body massage, including genitals and breasts, feels natural. Other couples feel strange about purposefully staying at level 5 rather than proceeding to erotic flow. Most couples value playful touch, but others find sensual or erotic touch easier to integrate and don't engage in playful touch. We encourage you to enjoy nondemand pleasuring, both sensual and playful. Give yourself at least three opportunities to experiment with playful touch. If it's not the right fit for you, drop it. However, don't drop nondemand pleasuring.

Integrating intimacy/pleasuring/eroticism is motivating and empowering. All three dimensions count. Being receptive and responsive to touch and being touched is key to maintaining strong, resilient desire. Pleasuring is inviting, not demanding. Pleasuring facilitates variable, flexible sexuality—the scenario can include playful and erotic touch, or transition to intercourse. Openness to these sexual dimensions enhances anticipation, the key to desire.

Leslie and Donovan

Leslie and Donovan became a couple their junior year of college. Leslie was a highly motivated, diligent student while Donovan, although smart, was easily distracted by computer and video games. They began as a romantic love/passionate sex/idealized (limerance) couple. There was lots of pleasuring as well as intercourse and orgasm. Leslie was very pleased with her desire/pleasure/eroticism/satisfaction response.

Donovan joined ROTC as a means to pay tuition. When he was on weekend trainings or a six-week Navy program, Leslie was acutely aware of missing both touching and intercourse.

When they graduated, they vowed to coordinate their life plans so they could remain a couple. Donovan had less control of his life since the Navy's training and deployment regimen had to be followed. Leslie's career plans involved working while pursuing a master's degree in public administration. This was a portable career which made being a Navy wife a viable life organization. Pleasuring and sexuality was a powerful motivating and bonding factor.

We are fans of the romantic love/passionate sex/idealized phase, but it is fragile and time-limited. Commonly, the first element disrupted is idealization. In her work and classes, Leslie met men who were more focused and goal-oriented than Donovan. She enjoyed the attention and flirting. Donovan was jealous, especially of physically fit men who were financially successful. Arguments over other men were a source of stress. These arguments reduced Leslie's respect for Donovan, but not her trust in him and their relationship. Leslie was aware of the difference between a "crush" and an actual affair. She accepted that Donovan masturbated using porn when they were apart and saw no problem in that. Leslie masturbated to images of attractive men. She understood the boundary between fantasy and real-life behavior.

The incident which caused a crisis occurred on a training mission. Donovan had sex with prostitutes and acquired chlamydia. He ignored the symptoms and Leslie and Donovan were sexual when he returned. Four months later during a routine gynecological visit she had an STI screen and learned she had contracted chlamydia. Both physically and emotionally, Leslie felt betrayed. The gynecologist said Donovan needed to be tested and insisted they be treated at the same time. Otherwise, they would pass chlamydia back and forth. The physician emphasized that STI is a health/medical issue, not a moral judgment.

Donovan was embarrassed and remorseful; he did not want their relationship to end because of an STI. However, the romantic love/passionate sex/idealization phase was over. The question was how to build a new trust bond and develop a couple sexual style. In retrospect, Leslie wished they'd had the fidelity/monogamy discussion a year earlier. When she speaks to girlfriends and her younger sister she offers two pieces of advice based on primary prevention principles. First, in developing a couple sexual style after the limerance phase, emphasize the core role of nondemand pleasuring. Second, do not assume—have a clear discussion about fidelity and monogamy. Leslie and Donovan committed to a satisfying, secure, and sexual relationship which would lead to marriage. Each maintained autonomy in their lives, friendships, masturbation, and fantasy. However, emotional and sexual secrets involving other partners were not acceptable. Monogamy agreements respect autonomy but confront secrets which are harmful to the partner and relationship (McCarthy & Wald, 2013).

They chose the Complementary couple sexual style, the most common decision. Leslie and Donovan valued intimacy and eroticism and couple sexuality focused on desire and satisfaction. Leslie emphasized the value of nondemand pleasuring which reinforced their attachment bond. Pleasure is valuable whether it leads to intercourse or not. She wanted Donovan to genuinely embrace pleasuring, not placate her or be "politically correct." For Leslie, sensual and playful touching facilitated desire and feeling desirable. She thought of herself as the poster woman for "responsive sexual desire." About half the time this transitioned to intercourse. Leslie particularly enjoyed intercourse when Donovan took his time, so she experienced erotic flow before beginning intercourse. She valued playful dates and was pleased Donovan joined in rather than feel frustrated about intercourse. With this approach there was more pleasuring and more intercourse. Donovan was genuinely present and involved. Although Leslie wished Donovan had not been sexual with prostitutes and given her chlamydia, building a strong trust bond and couple sexual style reinforced the healing process. Nondemand pleasuring was more genuine than in the limerance phase. This enhanced Leslie's sexual desire and confidence. Leslie has great memories of the limerance phase, but the present integration of intimacy/pleasuring/eroticism feels more solid.

Every three months Leslie and Donovan planned a nondemand pleasuring date with a prohibition on intercourse and orgasm. She looked forward to these dates as an opportunity to experiment with new techniques, lotions, and music. Leslie attended yoga as well as mindfulness classes. She incorporated these techniques into their pleasuring dates. This ensured she and Donovan did not fall into the trap of routine, mechanical sex. Leslie valued variable, flexible couple sexuality. Donovan enjoyed nondemand pleasuring as an integral component in their sexual repertoire.

Keeping the Demand Out

The challenge is to ensure that the "demand" stays out of nondemand pleasuring. This is a couple task, not for you alone. When you say, "I need you to show that you want me" or he says, "You turned me on, you need to let me inside you," this can put you back in the intercourse or nothing power struggle. Nondemand pleasuring affirms that couple sexuality is about requests, sharing pleasure, and a positive influence process. Demands cause power struggles because the message is if you don't comply there will be negative consequences. Requests do not involve threats.

The time to talk about sexual issues is the day before being sexual. Don't do something that intimidates your partner or undermines the intimate team. Each person commits to keeping the demand out and agrees that even if frustrated or hurt you will not pressure or put down your partner. Stay connected as intimate and erotic friends. A strength of nondemand pleasuring is it invites you to freely experience sensual and playful touch without fear of pressure or negative consequences.

The distinction between requests and demands is crucial. A request says, "I am your sexual friend; this will enhance my pleasure." A demand says, "You need to do this for me and if you don't there will be big problems." Demands say there is only one option; requests involve awareness that there are many ways to share pleasure. You need not fear negative consequences if something doesn't work. Requests facilitate intimacy and pleasuring, demands create anticipatory and performance anxiety (Metz & Epstein, 2002). You owe it to yourself, your partner, and your relationship to keep the demand out and reinforce pleasuring.

Exercise: Sensual Pleasuring

Non-genital pleasuring (also called sensate focus) is a core technique to build comfort with giving and receiving touch. Traditionally, couples use the giver—receiver format. At a later time, you can experiment with mutual touching. Find the best fit for you.

The focus of sensual pleasuring is exploring feelings/sensations of 1–3 subjective arousal. When you use the giver—receiver format, let the woman be giver first. Engage in the type of sensual touch you enjoy giving rather than trying to second guess what he wants. He lies on his stomach, so you can explore the entire back of his body from the top of his head to the soles of his feet. Use massage, stroking, tickling, one to two fingers or your whole hand. Be aware of your feelings rather than second guess his feelings. Do you enjoy giving long, slow, warm, rhythmic touching? What parts of his body feel most sensual? Do you enjoy playing with his hair, massaging neck muscles, caressing his back, scratching his arms, exploring his spine, stroking his buttocks, rubbing your hands over his legs and thighs? Enjoy tickling the soles of his feet. Look at the back of his body and be aware of the one, two, or three areas you particularly enjoy touching.

Help him turn over. Look at the entire front of his body, especially his breasts, testicles, and penis. Look, do not touch. Begin by touching his forehead, face, and neck. Feel free to kiss as well as touch. Stroke his chest using both hands and then experiment with one hand or two to three fingers. Do not touch his nipples but notice if there are changes as a result of pleasuring. How does it feel to massage his stomach, including playing with his belly button? Do you enjoy slow, rhythmic touching or do you prefer playful or seductive touch? As you look at (but don't touch) his testicles and penis, be aware of whether he is flaccid, semi-erect, or erect. Don't stare, but you have the right to visually inspect his genitals. For many women, this is the first time you allow yourself an explanatory look—be comfortable and take your time. How do you feel about massaging his inner thighs—either together or separately? Explore with your hands or use your tongue and lips. Move down his body as you explore his legs, shins, feet, and toes. As the giving partner, what sensations/feelings contribute to 1–3 level of subjective pleasure? Do you enjoy being the giving partner? Many women feel that because the man gets a spontaneous erection there is no reason for sensual touch, this is a mistake. Enjoy experimenting with sensual touch.

Switch roles. Be open to receiving sensual touch. For many, if not most, couples nondemand pleasuring is a new experience. Sensual touch is the foundation for sexual response. It has value for itself as a sexual experience, allowing you to bask in the 1–3 level of sensations/feelings. Being receptive and responsive to nondemand pleasuring is a totally different experience than "foreplay." The focus is sensual pleasure, not sexual arousal. In the desire/pleasure/eroticism/satisfaction mantra, pleasure is valued for itself not just as a bridge to arousal and intercourse. Rather than being passive, you are active, aware, and mindful of sensuality. Proceed at your pace, not his. He is your intimate sexual friend who enjoys sensuality for himself as well as facilitating sensual feelings/sensations in different parts of your body with different touches. Savor the experience. Are you more comfortable receiving on the front or back of your body? What types of touch on what body parts feel sensual? Do you feel desirable as he looks at your vulva and breasts without touching them? Do either you or he rush ahead, or can you genuinely accept nondemand sensual pleasuring?

Experiment with mutual give-and-take pleasuring. Women value this because it is less structured. Partner interaction arousal feels "natural." Be active whether receiving or giving; don't fall into the over learned passive role. Enjoy nondemand sensual pleasure.

Mutual touching is similar to a sensual dance where your receptivity reinforces your partner's receptivity. Sensuality is the foundation for sexual response and is an integral component of sexuality. Specifically, where in your body do you experience sensual response? Bask in sensual feelings and enjoy your partner's sensuality.

Exercise: Playful Touch

Nondemand pleasuring includes playful touch, involving sensations/feelings in the 4–5 range.

Playful touch is more challenging than sensual touch because it mixes genital and non-genital pleasuring. Embrace the playful dimension. We suggest you take the lead. It's your decision whether to utilize the giver—receiver format or the mutual touching format. When it's his turn, he chooses his preferred format.

Enjoy genital touch. Traditionally, women start with non-genital and transition to genital. What about starting genitally and transitioning to your favorite non-genital pleasuring technique or transitioning from non-genital to genital and then reintroducing non-genital pleasuring? Don't touch like you are following a cookbook recipe. Playful touch is meant to be variable, flexible, and creative. Embrace sensations/feelings at the 4–5 level. Take advantage of the temporary prohibition on intercourse and orgasm to savor the experience of playful touch.

How does it feel to explore his penis and testicles? Rather than the focus on arousal to orgasm, keep the focus on playful, nondemand pleasuring of his penis. His penis wants to be played with and you can enjoy touching with sensations/feelings of 4–5 subjective arousal. Enjoy his penis and erection rather than feeling pressured or intimidated.

Explore his testicles. Be aware of the differences in size and shape. Enjoy the experience of pleasuring his testicles. Breast touching is supposed to be erotic for women, but not men. Be open to touching and exploring his breasts with licking, stroking, kissing that you enjoy giving. Are his breasts responsive to touch? Play with his nipples with your fingers or tongue; remember to mix genital and non-genital touch and enjoy the sensations/feelings.

What do you feel when receiving playful pleasure? Be aware of the pleasuring process—contrast that with the passivity of foreplay where he is focused on turning you on. Be mindful and actively involve yourself in pleasure whether in the mutual give-and-take format or in the receiving role.

When do you feel receptive and responsive to receiving breast stimulation? Some women prefer slow, rhythmic stroking while others prefer playful or seductive touch. Many women find focused breast stimulation, especially manual or oral nipple stimulation, is a turn-off if you are not feeling receptive. Identify the type of breast stimulation which facilitates 4–5 subjective arousal. The message is do it your way, not give him power over your sexuality.

This is even more important when it involves vulva, clitoral, and vaginal touching. You have a right to your preferred genital scenario that involves mixing playful, seductive, and exploratory touch. This involves non-genital pleasuring rather than focused genital touch. Experiment with this two, three, or four times in adopting a playful, nondemand approach to genital pleasuring.

What is your favorite mix of genital and non-genital pleasuring? Where in your body do you savor the 4–5 sensations? Do you prefer mutual giving and receiving or taking turns? In what ways

> is playful touch different than sensual touch? In what ways is it different from "foreplay"? Embrace playful touch as integral to your sexual voice—a valuable sexual dimension.

The Mantra of Intimacy/Pleasuring/Eroticism

Affirm the mantra of intimacy/pleasuring/eroticism for yourself and your relationship. This reinforces your partner valuing broad-based couple sexuality. He gives up the traditional male focus on intercourse as a pass–fail test. Your experience with sensual and playful touch makes the pleasuring concept personal and concrete. Your enthusiasm is crucial, but not enough. Embrace the value of sensual and playful touch as an intimate sexual team. Pleasuring enhances desire, especially when valued for itself. Both partners are committed to ensure the demand element is confronted; don't allow it to creep in. Pleasuring and eroticism are very different dimensions, but not adversarial or incompatible. Pleasurable sensations/feelings can serve as a bridge to eroticism. Erotic scenarios usually transition to intercourse and orgasm. However, both partners embracing nondemand pleasuring as sexual and fulfilling in itself adds to your sexual repertoire. In the same manner, both partners embrace eroticism as valuable for itself, not just as a bridge to intercourse. Pleasuring/eroticism is a couple process. With intimacy/pleasuring/eroticism each component is valued and the whole is more than the component parts.

Summary

Nondemand pleasuring is an integral component of the desire/pleasure/eroticism/satisfaction mantra. Pleasuring involves sensual and playful touching with sensations/feelings in the 1–5 subjective arousal range. The key is to keep the demand out and accept pleasuring as valuable for itself rather than a mandate for intercourse and orgasm. Nondemand pleasuring can involve taking turns or mutual giving and receiving. Nondemand pleasuring is integral to couple sexuality. A powerful role is to reinforce the variable, flexible couple approach to sharing pleasure while confronting the individual sex performance model. Pleasuring can and does serve as a bridge to intercourse, but that is not a mandate nor is it the primary function. Pleasuring reinforces the variable, flexible approach to couple sexuality, while confronting the routine. mechanical expectation that all sexual touch must result in intercourse. Unpredictability and playfulness are particular strengths of nondemand pleasuring. Sexuality is much more than intercourse. Sensual and playful touch is an invaluable couple resource.

Both sensual and playful touch are integral dimensions of couple sexuality. Pleasuring is a bridge to eroticism, intercourse, and orgasm, but its chief function is to share pleasure.

7

INTEGRATED EROTICISM

Eroticism is the most controversial dimension of the desire/pleasure/eroticism/satisfaction mantra. There is more bad advice posted on internet sites on the topic of eroticism than almost any area of sexual function. Many women associate eroticism with male sexual misbehavior—porn, strip clubs, orgies, and prostitutes. Porn scenarios and fantasies are mistakenly assumed to be the essence of eroticism (Hamann, et al., 2004).

We take a totally different approach, advocating for integrated eroticism. Eroticism is best understood as a positive, integral component of the desire/pleasure/eroticism/satisfaction mantra. Eroticism is as much the domain of women as men. Eroticism is different than pleasuring—complementary, not adversarial or incompatible.

What are the key components of eroticism? Eroticism involves taking emotional and sexual risks, creativity and mystery, high levels of physical and emotional intensity, not being "socially desirable," and unpredictable sexual scenarios (Perel, 2006). In contrast, pleasuring is about warm, loving, predictable, mutual, comfortable, secure attachment. Eroticism is about energizing your relationship, taking risks, challenging boundaries, and reinforcing energy and vitality. Contrary to porn videos where the message is the wilder and more out of control the woman, the more erotic she is, integrated eroticism accepts that your erotic voice is integrated with your sexual voice. Embrace erotic scenarios and techniques which are the right fit for you rather than perform for the man or feel you have to prove yourself sexually.

Eroticism involves feelings/sensations of subjective arousal from 6–10 (5 is beginning arousal, 10 is orgasm). Orgasm is part of an erotic experience, but the core of eroticism is high intensity feelings/sensations. "Erotic flow" refers to levels 8 or 9 of subjective arousal. Orgasm is best understood as the natural continuation of erotic flow. Pleasuring/arousal/eroticism naturally flows to orgasm; but not orgasm as a pass–fail sex test.

There are three eroticism/arousal styles: (1) partner interaction arousal, (2) self-entrancement arousal, and (3) role enactment arousal. Partner interaction arousal is the most common. The focus is on partner responsivity, following the adage that the major aphrodisiac is an involved, aroused partner. This is the type of arousal shown in R-rated movies. Your partner's arousal is facilitated by your arousal, and his arousal facilitates your arousal. Focus on mutuality, giving and receiving pleasurable and erotic touch.

Self-entrancement arousal involves taking turns giving and receiving touch, similar to the format of sensate focus exercises. The receiving partner takes in pleasure, allowing sensual and sexual feelings/sensations to build. The giving partner is aroused by the receiving partner's arousal. Use of self-entrancement arousal increases with aging. Partners usually take turns giving and receiving, although asynchronous sexual experiences are also valued. The receiving partner is active, not passive—you're mindful and accepting of erotic sensations/feelings.

Role enactment arousal involves incorporating external resources into couple sexuality. This can include X-rated videos, sexual toys (paddle, ropes, handcuffs, clips, blindfold), sharing an erotic fantasy, or playing out a BDSM scenario. Internet and "expert" advice advocates for role enactment arousal.

Many marital therapists reject role enactment arousal as anti-intimate. Role enactment arousal emphasizes sexual risk-taking and creating an erotic charge but is not anti-intimacy.

All three arousal styles facilitate eroticism. However, not all arousal styles fit all couples. The great majority of couples utilize partner interaction arousal and a significant number utilize self-entrancement arousal, at least on occasion. Many couples experiment with role enactment arousal.

For some, it is their preferred erotic style. Others discard role enactment arousal or only use it on special occasions. The Emotionally Expressive couple sexual style is most compatible with role enactment arousal. The Best Friend and Traditional couple sexual styles typically reject role enactment arousal.

The key is integrating your arousal/eroticism style into desire/pleasure/eroticism/satisfaction. As with other aspects of sexuality, "one size never fits all." Rather than a "right/wrong," the issue is how to integrate eroticism into your sexual relationship. Specifically, how does your "erotic voice" promote sexual anticipation, subjective and objective arousal, and feeling satisfied as a sexual woman and couple. Eroticism is integrated with your feelings and preferences to create strong, resilient sexual desire. Your erotic scenarios are as important as his. Your right to veto an erotic scenario is crucial with confidence that your partner will honor your veto. Having the right to say "no" gives you the power to say "yes" to the type of eroticism which is the right fit for you. Contrary to myths of unbridled lust or sex without boundaries, integrated eroticism is about choice of erotic scenarios and techniques. Finding an erotic voice which fits your feelings and preferences is empowering. The mandate to prove yourself erotically or perform for your partner is intimidating and negates desire.

Erotic Fantasies

If you fantasize about sex with your brother-in-law or being gang-raped does this mean that's what you really want? Are fantasies the x-ray which reveals hidden sexual desires? Are you (and everyone else) sexually perverse?

Sexual fantasy and real-life sexual behavior are very different dimensions. By its nature, erotic fantasies are socially unacceptable. The most common erotic fantasies are sex with an inappropriate partner (boss, neighbor, minister, movie star), forced sex or being forced, watching someone being sexual or being watched, or sex with someone of the same gender. In the great majority of cases erotic fantasy and real-life sex are totally separate (McCarthy, 2015). What gives the fantasy an erotic charge is that it's different than real-life couple behavior. When couples play out an erotic fantasy, a common outcome is it's a sexual "dud." Acting it out robs the fantasy of its erotic charge. Erotic fantasies make better fantasy than real sexual behavior.

An example is a common male fantasy of women fighting to orally stimulate him. The fantasy of three women sexually eager to service the man can be highly charged, but if played out the outcome is increased self-consciousness, awkwardness, and feeling sexually intimidated.

Being sexually forced or coerced by one or more men is a common female fantasy. Being taken over sexually is a powerful fantasy. In reality, rape is aversive and traumatic. The erotic charge comes from the forbidden fantasy, not the desire for a real-life experience.

Fantasy and reality are totally different domains. Erotic fantasy is a sexually charged sixth dimension (gear). Give yourself permission to use erotic fantasies as a bridge to sexual desire and a bridge to erotic flow and orgasm. Erotic fantasies are the most common form of multiple stimulation during partner sex (Nelson, 2012). You are free to use erotic fantasies how and when you like without feeling self-conscious or guilty. Erotic fantasies enhance your sexual presence. The healthy role of fantasy is to facilitate eroticism and add vitality to your sexual experience.

In the great majority of cases verbally sharing the erotic fantasy is a self-defeating strategy no matter what internet sex sites advise. Sharing the erotic fantasy increases self-consciousness. There is nothing more anti-erotic than self-consciousness.

It is a challenge to integrate eroticism into your couple sexual style, but a challenge worth meeting. Eroticism is integral to healthy female and couple sexuality.

Anna and Regis

Anna was 38 when she found her genuine adult sexual voice. She graduated college at 22, married at 28, had her first child at 31, and her last child at 34. As a woman Anna felt good about her personal, professional, marital, and family life, but not her sex life. Sex was functional, but routine and not energizing. Anna "loved Regis but did not feel in love with him." She'd recently read "Mating in Captivity" (Perel, 2006) and realized she'd not only de-eroticized Regis, but de-eroticized herself. Was an affair the answer for the lost part of Anna?

Anna remembered her college years as new and exciting as she learned about herself, the world, relationships, and sexuality. She had special memories of romantic love/passionate sex dating relationships where her desire was high. Anna prided herself in using contraception and practicing safe sex. Sexuality was a special, energizing dimension of her young adult life. What happened to the sexually enthusiastic Anna? She still felt pro-sexual, but sex with Regis was disappointing and infrequent.

Anna valued her life—parenting, career, marriage, religious beliefs, community involvement, extended family, and friends. Although challenging, she felt good about this balance in her life. Her walking group, book club, dinner parties, trips with other families contributed to the quality of her life. The missing piece was her sex life. Rather than sexuality having a 15–20% role of energizing the marriage and reinforcing feelings of desire and desirability, Anna felt sex was dull and mechanical.

Anna envied a female friend who had initiated her divorce two years ago and was enjoying being the sought-after woman. Anna knew Regis loved her and was committed to their family but missed the excitement of romantic love/passionate sex. There was a consultant at work who was a well-known "womanizer." Anna fantasized about beginning a "fun affair." He was an attractive, funny man who enjoyed flirting and was open to a "fling." Anna wrestled with the impact of an affair on her, Regis, their marriage, and family.

Anna wanted a satisfying and secure marriage and was afraid an affair would disrupt her long-term life goals. However, the short-term drama and excitement was alluring. Anna was neither naive nor moralistic—she had observed the highs and lows of affairs through her friends and colleagues' experiences. Anna wanted the erotic charge of an affair, but not the pain it would cost Regis, her family, and herself.

After a contentious business meeting Anna, the consultant, and three colleagues went to "happy hour." Anna was very aware of the tingling feelings elicited by his flirtatious touch and her fantasy of sneaking off to a hotel. Anticipation and erotic feelings were strong. Erotic fantasy is all about illicit sex. A second drink could facilitate the mood, but since she had to drive home Anna passed on the drink, but not on the seductive feelings.

That night as she was showering, Anna mentally played out an erotic encounter with the consultant. As she got into bed the fantasy served as a bridge to desire and she and Regis had a very erotic encounter. This provided a valuable insight—Anna could use an erotic fantasy as a bridge to enhance marital sex. Even more important, she could create erotic scenarios with Regis which enhanced feelings of desire and desirability. In truth, the mind is your major sex organ. Anna had not taken advantage of her "erotic voice," wanting it to come "naturally" rather than using erotic fantasy to enhance desire. An erotic key for Anna was anticipation and unpredictability. She had not used these techniques to enhance sexual quality, partly out of lethargy and partly because of the belief she shouldn't need to. Anna had felt self-conscious about erotic fantasy, especially of other partners. She gave herself permission to utilize erotic fantasies and scenarios to give marital sexuality a special charge. There are many ways to integrate eroticism for you as a woman and in your relationship. This was the right fit for Anna as a 38-year-old married woman.

Embracing Eroticism

The challenge for the sexually healthy woman is not just to accept, but to embrace eroticism. Eroticism is a positive, integral component of female sexuality. Integrate your "erotic voice" with couple sexuality rather than feel pressured or intimidated by your partner's concept of eroticism, the "hot" media messages, or the porn model. Incorporate erotic scenarios and techniques that fit you. You don't have to prove anything to your partner or anyone else.

The majority of women feel intimidated and put off by erotic suggestions provided by the media and sex sites. The technique of verbally sharing erotic fantasies, playing out BDSM scenarios, watching porn videos during sex, or swinging from the chandelier make better fantasy than real-life couple sexuality. What kind of partner-interaction, self-entrancement, and/or role-enactment scenarios enhance eroticism for you? Eroticism is yet another example that "sexually, one size never fits all." You do not have to prove you are sexually free. What provides a unique erotic charge for you? Embracing eroticism gives you the freedom and power to decide how best to use erotic fantasies. For most women, this means keeping them as private fantasies. For those who choose to experiment with verbally sharing fantasies or behaviorally acting them out, make sure it is the right fit for you. Rather than pressure to "do the right thing," what is right for you? Performance pressure subverts sexual desire. Freedom and choice promotes healthy eroticism and sexuality. Some types of eroticism are anti-intimate, but erotic strategies and techniques are applicable to couple sexuality.

A common issue with eroticism involves anal stimulation generally and anal intercourse specifically. Your anal area has a number of nerve endings which promote erotic sensations. Many women find manual anal or buttock stimulation highly erotic. For others anal stimulation has an "unclean" or even perverse connotation which overrides positive sensations and feelings.

Anal intercourse has a strong erotic charge for many men (others find it a turn-off). Is being anally penetrated erotic for you or do you do it for your partner? Comfort and enjoyment with anal stimulation generally and anal intercourse specifically requires high arousal and a lubricant. Without arousal and an additional lubricant anal penetration can be painful. When the partner is aware of your feelings, uses a lubricant as part of the pleasuring/eroticism process, and slowly guides insertion some women experience anal intercourse as highly erotic, especially when she also engages in self-pleasuring of her clitoral area. Other women find it acceptable, but more enjoyable for him than for you. Other women find anal intercourse anti-erotic. Like everything else sexually, the question is what is the right fit for you in terms of pleasure and eroticism.

More women feel responsive to manual anal stimulation than anal intercourse. Some women are comfortable both giving and receiving anal stimulation while others only enjoy receiving, especially at high levels of erotic flow. We advocate integrated eroticism which accepts your unique feelings and preferences. Embracing eroticism is about accepting and expanding, not performing or proving yourself. Feel motivated and empowered, not intimidated.

> **Exercise: Developing Erotic Scenarios**
>
> This exercise is about sexual freedom and power. You have the right to erotic scenarios and techniques that allow you to feel subjective arousal of 6–10. Eroticism is not the man's domain; it is equally your domain. You have the right to develop erotic scenarios that are a special fit for you. Your partner has the right to veto scenarios which are intimidating or a turn-off for him, and trust that you will not coerce or punish him. Assume he is open to your requests. Don't second guess him or worry about his reaction. It is his responsibility to say "no."
>
> The key to developing erotic scenarios is to focus on what promotes intense sexual feelings/sensations for you, not for him. Take emotional and sexual risks, don't worry about being "socially acceptable." You don't need anybody's approval, nor do you need to prove yourself. Identify erotically inviting scenarios and techniques and give yourself permission to play these out.
>
> Traditionally, women have been more comfortable with scenarios and techniques that promoted intimacy, nondemand pleasuring, and playful touch. However, you gave up your sexual freedom and power when eroticism, intercourse, and orgasm came into play. You followed the man's scenario driven by his erection and desire for orgasm. This is the time to challenge that traditional pattern.
>
> The majority of women find that giving and receiving sensual and playful touch is much superior to traditional "foreplay" where you are passive and it's his job to get you ready for intercourse. When subjective arousal is 5, how do you transition from pleasuring to eroticism? Is partner-interaction, self-entrancement, or role enactment arousal most inviting? Go with your feelings and preferences, not what "should" be erotic or his preference. Do you view

his erection as an affirmation of sexual pleasure and playfulness or as pressure to hurry up and get aroused? If you feel pressure, what can you do to slow down the process and focus on your erotic feelings and sensations? Pleasure and eroticism are core sexual dimensions.

A key to eroticism is to stay focused on sensations/feelings, not treat sex as a performance or competition. With partner interaction arousal you piggy-back your arousal on his (stay focused on your subjective arousal). Many women prefer self-entrancement arousal because it allows you to focus on erotic feelings and sensations and be "sexually selfish." The difference between self-entrancement arousal and foreplay is that rather than the man being in charge with the goal of intercourse, you are in charge and follow your rhythm of pleasure and eroticism, which may or may not flow to intercourse.

Establish at least one (and up to three) partner interaction arousal scenarios. Then at least one (and up to three) self-entrancement scenarios.

Developing your unique erotic voice gives you the freedom to experiment with subjective arousal scenarios.

Partner Interaction Arousal/Eroticism

Common partner interaction scenarios are being sexual outside the bed room (family room, guest bedroom, living room), dressing in an attractive outfit or semi-clothed; you taking the sexual lead; choreographing the rhythm of kissing, touching, and stroking which reflects your level of subjective arousal; giving and receiving manual and oral stimulation; he turned on by your erotic flow to orgasm whether with manual, oral, or rubbing stimulation; he verbalizing how sexy you are; transitioning to intercourse at your initiation—use your favorite position and type of thrusting; you set the rhythm of thrusting; give yourself permission to use erotic fantasies during intercourse—including fantasies of multiple partners, being dominant, being sexually forced.

In reinforcing your sexual desire it's important that the transition from pleasuring to eroticism to intercourse be your call. Ideally, intercourse is anticipated by both partners, and both are free to initiate and guide intromission. Increase involvement with intercourse rather than mechanical in and out thrusting. Experiment with long, slow thrusting, circular thrusting, he controls thrusting, you control thrusting, up and down thrusting, playful thrusting. Experiment with side-by-side intercourse; woman on-top; rear-entry; you sitting, he kneeling; he on top, you putting your feet on his shoulders; standing intercourse; switching intercourse positions. Experiment with multiple stimulation during intercourse—clitoral stimulation with your fingers while he sucks on your breast; you giving testicle stimulation while he rubs your buttocks; passionately kissing while enjoying circular thrusting; switch intercourse positions three times ending with deep thrusting from the rear-entry position while you are orgasmic using clitoral stimulation; standing in front of a mirror and enjoying visual feedback with your legs around him as he thrusts.

A key to partner interaction arousal/eroticism is that your erotic response plays off your partner's. Partner interaction arousal multiplies the effect of your arousal and enhances erotic flow. Although some women prefer one focused erotic touch, the majority enjoy multiple stimulation during partner interaction arousal. Do not shut down your erotic response and preferences. Your eroticism is just as important as his.

Self-Entrancement Arousal/Eroticism

Self-entrancement arousal grows in popularity as couples age. Pleasuring exercises demonstrate that self-entrancement arousal is relevant at any age. You are in charge with a focus on feelings and sensations rather than being passive. The foreplay scenario causes self-consciousness, and nothing is more anti-erotic than self-consciousness. Be actively involved in the eroticism process.

With self-entrancement arousal you usually take turns giving and receiving, but this is not a mandate. Many women genuinely enjoy the giving role and are turned-on by your power to activate erotic response. Most women find it erotic to be the receiving partner and relish pleasuring/eroticism/erotic flow to orgasm. The key is to actively involve yourself with erotic sensations and feelings rather than passively receiving stimulation. Do not feel pressured to perform.

Develop an erotic scenario (s) being the receiving partner and an erotic scenario (s) being the giving partner.

A common receiving self-entrancement arousal scenario involves beginning with mutual pleasuring. When your subjective arousal is 4–5 transition to the receiving role. Be relaxed, mindful, open to playful and erotic touch. Request/guide him in pleasuring you. He mixes the type and rhythm of touching and stroking. Sexual arousal and erotic response is facilitated by unpredictable feelings and sensations. When erotic flow is 8–9, focused rhythmic stimulation allows you to flow from eroticism to orgasm.

Openness and mindfulness are the core characteristics of the receiving partner. Embrace being saturated with pleasure; emotionally and physically open your body to eroticism. Most women find genital stimulation is not erotic unless subjective arousal is 4 or 5. Are you open to breast stimulation with his hands, mouth, or penis? Do you prefer genital kisses or have him suck on your breasts, skin, vulva, or thighs? Do you respond to oral stimulation (cunnilingus)? What type of stimulation allows you to go from 6–9? Do you enjoy teasing, seductive touch; rubbing his penis against your buttocks or breasts; receiving manual or oral stimulation; being relaxed and mindful; feeling surrounded by pleasure and erotic sensations?

Erotic flow to orgasm (transitioning from 9 to 10) is special with self-entrancement arousal. Rather than feeling self-conscious and working to orgasm, allow yourself to go with the erotic flow which naturally culminates in orgasm. The majority of women value multiple stimulation, although a significant minority respond to one focused stimulation. During multiple stimulation, be open to manual and oral stimulation, give yourself permission to use a "socially unacceptable" erotic fantasy, move your pelvis rhythmically, and/or verbalize "I love this—I'm going to come." The single focus woman uses manual, oral, or rubbing stimulation to let go and be orgasmic.

In giving self-entrancement arousal, a common scenario is being turned-on by your power to elicit erotic response from your partner. Whether manual or oral stimulation, transitioning to intercourse at high levels of erotic flow or continuing erotic stimulation to orgasm, own your erotic power. You control his transition from pleasure to arousal to erotic flow to orgasm. An advantage of giving self-entrancement arousal is that it is your choice of erotic scenarios and techniques. This reinforces being a desirable, valued sexual woman.

Role Enactment Arousal/Eroticism

This is the most controversial arousal/eroticism style and the one emphasized on the internet, media sources, and by "sex experts." Don't let yourself feel pressured or intimidated. Role enactment scenarios are a choice, not a mandate. You don't need to prove eroticism. Role enactment arousal is most compatible with the Emotionally Expressive couple sexual style, and least acceptable for the Traditional and Best Friend styles. Some Complementary sexual style couples enjoy role enactment arousal, but just as many, if not more, find it is not the right fit. Some couples use role enactment scenarios on occasion for a special erotic charge, but usually utilize partner interaction and self-entrancement arousal. The bottom line is that like everything sexually, role enactment arousal/eroticism is a choice—one size never fits all.

Common role enactment scenarios include watching an X-rated video as a sexual warm-up, playing sex games with ropes and blindfolds, engaging in a triadic sex scenario including simultaneous anal and vaginal penile penetration, playing out an erotic fantasy of an older man and an adolescent virgin, you as a dominatrix with him as a sexual slave catering to your every sexual whim, being sexual in front of a mirror and watching erotic flow build, reading a favorite erotic passage from a book or poem, tying your partner up and rubbing your body against him to orgasm.

Highly charged erotic fantasies usually do not translate to real-life eroticism. When played out they turn into sexual "duds." Role enactment arousal needs to retain an erotic charge when played out. An example is erotic feelings generated by being prevented from having an orgasm even though you are highly stimulated. A negative example is a male fantasy of three women sexually servicing him which feels awkward and non-arousing for both the man and woman when played out.

A key to role enactment arousal is the ability to enact a "non-socially acceptable" scenario without self-consciousness.

A core guideline is each partner has the right to veto or stop a scenario. Trust the partner will honor your veto without judgment or put-downs. Freedom, choice, and risk-taking energizes role enactment arousal; needing to prove something to the partner subverts role enactment eroticism. Couples who enjoy role enactment arousal have a powerful erotic resource.

Summary

Eroticism is an integral component of the desire/pleasure/eroticism/satisfaction mantra. Eroticism is the most controversial dimension and can be misused in an anti-intimate manner. Integrated eroticism is healthy for the woman, man, and couple. Although a different dimension from pleasuring, eroticism is integral to the pleasuring/eroticism/erotic flow/orgasm process. You have the right to your erotic voice with preferences for scenarios and techniques. Eroticism promotes emotional and sexual risk-taking, creativity, mystery, intense sensations, unpredictability, and sexual vitality. You have the right to choose partner-interaction, self-entrancement, and/or role enactment arousal/eroticism. Eroticism is about embracing a vital, intense sexuality which energizes your bond.

8

SATISFACTION: MORE THAN ORGASM

Most men (and women) believe "orgasm=satisfaction." Although we are strong advocates for female orgasm, it is crucial to understand that satisfaction is more than orgasm. In the desire/pleasure/eroticism/satisfaction mantra, satisfaction is the second most important dimension. Satisfaction involves feeling good about yourself as a sexual woman and bonded and energized as a sexual couple. This includes being orgasmic, but not orgasm as an individual pass–fail sex test. Orgasm is a natural continuation of the pleasuring/eroticism process (Graham, 2014).

Orgasm is a positive, integral component of female sexuality, integral to your "erotic voice." Female orgasmic response is first class, not inferior to the predictable, stereotypic male orgasm. The man has one orgasm during intercourse, accompanied by ejaculation. The most common male sex dysfunction is premature ejaculation—he reaches orgasm in less than two minutes and does not feel in control of when he ejaculates. In contrast, female orgasmic response is characterized by variability, flexibility, complexity, and individual differences. Female orgasm is first class, not inferior to male orgasm.

The core issue is acceptance of your "orgasmic voice." Female orgasmic patterns are quite individualistic. Only one in six women have the same orgasmic pattern as men—a single orgasm during intercourse without additional stimulation. One in three women are never or almost never orgasmic during intercourse. Her orgasmic pattern involves erotic techniques—manual, oral, rubbing, or vibrator stimulation. This is not a sex dysfunction; it is a normal, healthy orgasmic pattern (Heiman &

LoPiccolo, 1988). Two out of three women can be orgasmic during intercourse. The key strategies are transitioning to intercourse at high levels of erotic flow and multiple stimulation during intercourse.

Be aware that 15–18% of women have a multi-orgasmic response pattern. Two to three percent experience an emission occurring during orgasm. Only 10–15% of women are orgasmic 90% or more during couple sex. What these data illustrate are individual differences in women's orgasmic patterns. Orgasmic differences are accepted and honored. Unfortunately, in the culture and media, there is a destructive tendency to highlight a performance-oriented "right" orgasmic response whether G-spot, tantric, deep vaginal, hour-long, multiple orgasms, or whatever the new orgasm fad is. Pressure for the "right" orgasm is intimidating. The message is you're not "good enough." Orgasm is not an individual performance goal. Orgasm is the natural continuation of the pleasuring/eroticism process, not an individual performance test. You are responsible for your orgasm. Sexually, the couple are intimate and erotic allies who value your orgasmic voice. Accepting your orgasmic pattern(s) is key for sexual satisfaction. You don't need to perform for your partner or meet some arbitrary criterion for the "perfect" orgasm. From the foundation of acceptance choose whether to enhance your orgasmic voice. Don't fall into the trap of feeling inferior or second-class. The major cause of secondary female sexual interest/arousal disorder (FSIAD) and secondary non-orgasmic response is the performance pressure caused by believing you are deficit and need to perform the "right" way. Healthy sexuality is about acceptance and satisfaction, not performing for your partner or meeting an arbitrary performance goal.

Orgasm is an integral component of female sexuality. The average woman is orgasmic during 70% of couple sexual encounters (Ter Kulie, Both, & van Lankveld, 2012). There are occasions where she feels more satisfied with the experience than her partner even though he was orgasmic, and she wasn't. If sex were just about orgasm, women (and men) would masturbate rather than engage in couple sex. Masturbation is a reliable way to reach orgasm. By its nature, couple sexuality is variable and flexible with a range of roles, meanings, and outcomes. Sometimes satisfaction is about feeling bonded, other times sharing pleasure, a tension reducer, a way to reinforce attraction, soothing after a career or family disappointment, to end a period of alienation, to conceive a baby, or to heal after an argument. Satisfaction can involve a number of emotional and physical needs, especially feeling desire and desirable. Sometimes you want an orgasm, other times you want a hug. Sometimes the experience involves lust and intensity; other times a sensual and playful connection. The core of satisfaction is feeling good about yourself as a sexual woman and energized and special as a sexual couple.

Afterplay

Afterplay is the most ignored sexual phase. Afterplay enhances personal and sexual satisfaction. Rather than the traditional two—three-minute cuddling, "I love you," and then sleep, we suggest developing personally inviting afterplay scenarios. This could include an intimate scenario of sharing emotions and acknowledging the specialness of your relationship, a playful scenario, showering together, disclosing sensitive material from your family or childhood, a sensual massage or back rub, making a pot of tea or having a glass of wine, or sharing hopes/dreams.

Most women emphasize afterplay to share intimacy, but this is not true all the time. Leave room for fun, creative, silly, or irreverent experiences. Create two, three, or four afterplay scenarios which feel special and bonding. Not all sexuality needs to be intimate, mutual, and serious. Sexual play can be part of the mix. Afterplay enhances emotional and sexual satisfaction.

Dealing with Mediocre, Dissatisfying, or Dysfunctional Sexual Encounters

The sex positive approach to female and couple sexuality is a dominant theme of this book. Desire/pleasure/eroticism/satisfaction affirms the 15–20% role and value of sexuality. It is important to acknowledge that occasional mediocre, dissatisfying, or dysfunctional sexual encounters occur with even the healthiest and most sex positive women and couples. Rather than panic, guilt, or blame, be aware that negative sexual experiences do not negate sexual satisfaction. In fact, a measure of healthy female sexuality is to turn toward your partner rather than away from him when there is a problematic sexual encounter. This is easier when the man has a dysfunctional experience—whether low desire, loss of erection, premature ejaculation, or ejaculatory inhibition. Whether once a month, once every ten times, or once a year, this happens to almost all men. If the sex problem is chronic, it needs to be addressed in couple therapy. However, mediocre, dissatisfying, or dysfunctional encounters are a normal part of variable, flexible, male, female, and couple sexuality. He is a sexual man, not a perfectly functioning sex machine. Turn toward him as his intimate and erotic friend. Regroup and be sexual in the next few days when you are receptive and responsive to giving and receiving pleasure-oriented touching.

What about when sex is dissatisfying or dysfunctional for you? This is normal, not a symptom of sex dysfunction. Feeling guilty or apologizing is anti-erotic, as well as unnecessary. You can voice disappointment, but do not feel like a sexual failure nor shameful about sexuality. Self-acceptance involves both strengths and vulnerabilities. Sexual self-esteem is not contingent on everything being perfect. Don't deny dissatisfying or dysfunctional sexual experiences. Acknowledge these without apologizing.

Is this a normal "blip" or a sexual problem which needs to be attended to? Can the problem be resolved, modified, or worked around so that it doesn't control couple sexuality? Turn toward your partner. He is your sexual friend, not someone you apologize to, perform for, or prove something to.

Desire, arousal, and orgasm are inherently variable and flexible. Interestingly, this becomes increasingly true of men after 40 or 50. Acceptance of variable sexuality is a major challenge for the man and couple. Typically, male desire and response is very predictable in his 20s and 30s. This reinforces the traditional mistaken view that male sex is superior. In the long term, especially with couples over 40 or 50, the variable, flexible Good Enough Sex (GES) approach promotes satisfying sexuality. The individual sex performance model leads to frustration, embarrassment, and avoidance. Rather than panicking or apologizing, you and your partner accept GES, including occasional mediocre, dissatisfying, or dysfunctional encounters. Generally, women find accepting GES as the right fit much easier than men do.

Lisa and Blake

Like most couples, Lisa and Blake began as a romantic love/passionate sex/idealized couple (limerance phase). They had fond memories of erotic highs and satisfaction during those first 16 months. However, like many couples, they did not transition to a couple sexual style. Instead sex became problematic, especially after the birth of their two children. The pattern was even more problematic when the children were adolescents. They look back on the 22 years of their marriage with fond memories, but also a number of regrets, especially sexual regrets. In the "couple again" phase, they have an opportunity to develop a new couple sexual style which promotes desire/pleasure/eroticism/satisfaction. They are committed to getting it right, especially enhanced relational and sexual satisfaction. For 70% of couples, sexual satisfaction goes down at the birth of their first child and doesn't go up again until the last child leaves home. The "empty nest" syndrome is a misnomer. The "couple again" phase is one of revitalized desire and satisfaction (McCarthy & Pierpaoli, 2015).

Lisa and Blake want to enjoy this life phase. Rather than be stuck in regret or resentment, they focused on building a Complementary couple sexual style which promotes desire and satisfaction. They value both intimacy and eroticism; developed "her," "his," and "our" bridges to sexual desire; accept synchronous as well as asynchronous sexual experiences; integrate intimacy, pleasuring, and eroticism. They value GES and realize sexuality can have a range of roles, meanings, and outcomes. The best sex is mutual and synchronous, but they enjoy sexuality which is better for Lisa and other times better for Blake. With aging, they experience greater use of self-entrancement arousal/eroticism scenarios. Blake learned to "piggy-back" his arousal on Lisa's. She enjoys that they are erotic allies. Lisa wishes she'd been aware of this earlier, but now is committed to GES. She and Blake hope to share satisfying sexuality into their 60s, 70s, and 80s.

A key for sexual satisfaction is trust that Blake is her intimate sexual friend. This is important in sharing good times sexually and even more important in turning toward each other when sex is dissatisfying or dysfunctional. She trusts that emotionally and sexually "Blake has my back."

Accepting GES rather than demanding great sex each time is empowering. Lisa especially values experiences of responsive sexual desire where she feels freedom to stay with a sensual date, transition to mutually involving intercourse, enjoy a mutual erotic encounter, or Blake pleasuring her to orgasm. Freedom and choice enhance satisfaction. Their Complementary couple sexual style greatly reduced struggles over intercourse frequency. They have sex worth having rather than mediocre sex. Vibrancy and unpredictability add to sexual desire and satisfaction.

Contrary to when children were living at home, Lisa and Blake seldom have sex late at night. Although times to be sexual vary, late morning and sex after a nap are Lisa's favorites. Sexual encounters vary from three-minute "quickies" to two-hour lovemaking sessions. Unlike the past when lovemaking was under ten minutes, the majority of encounters are now 15–45 minutes, including five—seven minutes of intercourse. Lisa enjoys the mix and unpredictability more than Blake, but he agrees the longer scenarios are more satisfying. Although Blake strongly prefers transitioning to intercourse on his first erection, he's learned to accept the "wax and wane" of erection process rather than needing to rush to intercourse. They transition to intercourse at high levels of erotic flow rather than as soon as possible.

Multiple stimulation during intercourse adds to Lisa's erotic responsiveness. She feels free to utilize erotic fantasies during couple sex to enhance erotic flow. Lisa was aware that on average women are orgasmic 70% of encounters. In her younger years she was orgasmic 30–50% and is pleased that now she is orgasmic 80% of encounters. It is easier to be orgasmic with erotic stimulation, but on occasion she enjoys orgasm during intercourse (which is highly valued by Blake). Satisfaction is about acceptance and positive GES expectations.

Lisa and Blake value the couple again phase personally, relationally, and sexually. They do not treat sexuality with benign neglect. They are committed to growing as an intimate sexual couple who value desire/pleasure/eroticism/satisfaction. They look forward to vibrant, satisfying sexuality with aging.

Enhanced Sexual Satisfaction with Aging

Older couples report less sex frequency, but greater sexual satisfaction. In other words, arousal and orgasm are a challenge, but sexual satisfaction increases—often higher than in your 30s and 40s. You've "beaten the odds" and celebrate a resilient sexuality. Sex is more human, genuine, and you need each other in a way you hadn't in younger years. Couple sexuality is intimate and interactive, a sharing of pleasure and eroticism. Embrace being intimate and erotic allies. Enjoy that he needs your stimulation and sexual responsiveness in a way he hadn't 20 years ago. Mixing partner interaction arousal and self-entrancement arousal facilitates engagement and unpredictability. This variable, flexible approach to sexuality enhances desire and satisfaction. You are more of an intimate sexual team than in the past which increases bonding. Your active role in pleasuring and eroticism facilitates satisfaction. Although you might not have as attractive a body in terms of visual stimuli, this is more than made up for by engaging in give and take pleasuring and eroticism. Touching is the key for desire, not visual turn-on. Being active rather than passive facilitates sex and satisfaction. Satisfaction involves both process and outcome dimensions; this is clear with aging. Another dimension which becomes clear is the multiple roles, meanings, and outcomes of sexuality. Satisfaction is so much more than intercourse and orgasm. Sensual and playful sexuality is fulfilling. Asynchronous erotic scenarios using self-entrancement arousal increase with aging. Women enjoy self-entrancement arousal in both giving and receiving roles. In the receiving role you are active in orchestrating the sensations and feelings, welcoming erotic flow to orgasm. In the giving role, enjoy your power to pleasure him to orgasm. The variability, flexibility, and diversity of sexual scenarios contribute to satisfying sexuality. Valuing afterplay enhances satisfaction with aging.

Exercise: Enhancing Sexual Satisfaction

This exercise involves two categories—the sexual scenario itself and the afterplay scenario. Create first-class scenarios which enhance personal and couple satisfaction.

How can you set an inviting milieu? Is your preferred time to be sexual in the morning as soon as you wake? After a bath or shower? After a cup of coffee? Would you prefer to be sexual before or after lunch? What about before or after a nap? Before dinner (sex as an appetizer) or after dinner (sex as dessert)? Interestingly, few people prefer sex at the most common time—late at night. Sex is best when you are aware, awake, and open.

Do you prefer to initiate or for him to initiate, verbal or non-verbal, on the deck or in the bedroom, clothes on or off, with a glass of wine? Anticipation is a key to sexual desire. What kind of initiation enhances anticipation? Do you feel free to play out your chosen scenario? Are there external cues which enhance desire—lighting, candles, wine, a playful or seductive game?

Do you prefer the process of comfort, pleasure, arousal, eroticism, and transitioning to intercourse at high levels of erotic flow or do you have a different pleasure/eroticism pattern? Do you like spending time with sensual touching or do you prefer a quick transition to erotic touch? Do you respond best to partner interaction arousal, self-entrancement arousal, or role enactment arousal? Do you enjoy receiving stimulation, giving stimulation, or mutual stimulation? Are you most responsive to manual, oral, or rubbing stimulation?

Is intercourse part of your preferred sexual scenario? Who do you want to initiate intercourse? Do you like intercourse to begin as soon as possible or do you prefer a high level of erotic flow before transitioning to intercourse? What is your favorite intercourse position? What is your favorite type of thrusting? Do you enjoy multiple stimulation during intercourse? If intercourse is not part of your sexual repertoire, do you prefer manual, oral, rubbing, or vibrator stimulation?

What is your "orgasm voice"? Do you prefer being orgasmic before intercourse, during intercourse, or in afterplay? Don't be politically correct or do what your partner wants. This is your scenario—own it and play it out with your preferred sensations/feelings whether common or idiosyncratic. Accept your orgasmic pattern rather than feel it's not "perfect" or not the "right" type. If you want to change your orgasmic pattern it is easier to do so from a foundation of acceptance. Changes in your orgasmic voice are to enhance your satisfaction, not to prove something to your partner or meet a cultural expectation (based on unrealistic performance demands). An example is the woman who is multi-orgasmic with oral stimulation, but not orgasmic during intercourse. If orgasm during intercourse is a personally relevant goal, she can experiment with being orgasmic once or twice with oral stimulation and initiating the transition to intercourse at high levels of erotic flow. Utilize the woman on top position where he provides clitoral stimulation with his fingers as you guide the rhythm of circular thrusting and give yourself permission to enjoy an erotic fantasy of being seduced by your favorite musician. The key to orgasm during intercourse is transitioning at high levels of erotic flow and giving and receiving multiple stimulation during intercourse. If this enhances your orgasmic sensations/feelings own this new orgasmic scenario. It can be your preferred orgasmic pattern or to enjoy on special occasions. Other women are disappointed with the orgasmic feelings/sensations during intercourse, resulting in valuing her original orgasmic voice. Orgasm is an example of the adage, "sexually one size never fits all."

In designing your preferred scenario, the most important factor is developing couple sexuality which promotes satisfaction. Satisfaction involves reinforcing sexual self-esteem and feeling energized and bonded as a couple. Satisfaction includes encounters where you experience orgasm as well as accepting non-orgasmic experiences. A client cogently stated that at times "orgasm feels like an insignificant spasm while other times orgasm is a powerful validation of my being a sexual woman." Identify the sensations/feelings as well as the roles and meanings of orgasm and celebrate these.

Design afterplay scenarios which enhance satisfaction. The majority of afterplay experiences involve cuddling, "I love you," a kiss, and off to sleep. This is fine, but if it's the only afterplay scenario it loses specialness. We suggest each partner initiate at least one (and up to three) afterplay scenarios. These could include: (1) a playful scenario like tickling, playing a hand game on your partner's back, being "naughty"; (2) doing something active like bringing wine and dessert to bed or taking a shower together; (3) an emotionally meaningful scenario like recalling a time of closeness or planning an anniversary trip; (4) initiating a second sexual encounter; (5) talking about a sensitive issue from your personal or couple past; (6) planning a couple weekend getaway or requesting a special activity; (7) engaging in a nondemand pleasuring or playful scenario.

Find one, two, or three afterplay scenarios which allow you to feel special and bonded as a couple.

Non-Orgasmic Experiences and Satisfaction

What does it mean to be satisfied with a non-orgasmic encounter? Accept the inherent variability and flexibility of female and couple sexuality. A sexual encounter can be worthwhile and meaningful even though you are not orgasmic. This is core to GES and sexual satisfaction. The most anti-erotic thing your partner says is "Did you come?"

Many, in fact most, sexual experiences are asynchronous, i.e. desire/pleasure/eroticism/satisfaction is not equal. Enjoying your partner's pleasure and orgasm is healthy for you personally and as a couple. Be aware that there are sexual experiences where he is orgasmic, and you aren't, but the sex was more satisfying for you. Be aware of at least one experience where you felt special emotional satisfaction when not orgasmic.

Value mutual, synchronous sexual experiences where both share desire/pleasure/eroticism/satisfaction. However, you are setting yourself up for sexual dissatisfaction if that is the only acceptable outcome.

Embracing variable, flexible GES is key to sexual satisfaction. Accept the varied roles, meanings, and outcomes of sensual, playful, erotic, and intercourse sexuality. A key factor in satisfaction is turning toward your partner—accepting excellent and good sexual experiences as well as disappointing and dysfunctional experiences.

Increased Couple Satisfaction with Aging

Scientific data affirms that aging couples experience high sexual satisfaction (Hillman, 2008). This validates a broad-based couple approach to sharing pleasure. Women especially value sexuality and aging. When couples stop sex whether at 55, 65, 75, or 85 it is almost always the man's decision because he has lost confidence with erection, intercourse, and orgasm. He makes the decision unilaterally and conveys it non-verbally. He blames his partner for the cessation of sex which is unfair and unkind.

Two of three couples remain sexual in their 60s and one in three are sexual in their 70s (Laumann, Paik, & Rosen, 1999). What is the key to sexual desire and satisfaction with aging? Commonly, there are two components. First, you turn toward each other as intimate and erotic friends. The couple take to heart guidelines about female—male sexual equity; value intimacy, pleasuring, and eroticism; are intimate and erotic allies, including your partner "piggy-backing" his arousal on yours; embrace broad-based sexuality including nondemand pleasuring, playful touch, erotic scenarios and techniques, and multiple stimulation during intercourse; enjoy both synchronous and asynchronous sexuality; accept occasional dissatisfying or dysfunctional experiences. Female and couple sexuality come to fruition with the aging process. Sex during aging is genuine, human, meaningful, and healthy.

The second component is to accept GES with the focus on resilient desire, sharing pleasure, and enhancing satisfaction. GES is a triumph over the traditional male—female double standard and the myth of intercourse as an individual pass–fail test. GES recognizes that couple sexuality is inherently variable and flexible with a range of roles, meanings, and outcomes. The core of satisfaction is accepting the multiple motivations and feelings expressed as a couple. Sometimes sexuality is sharing intimate, sensual touch, other times a lustful, intense encounter. Often, the sexual scenario is asynchronous. Unlike in the 20s and 30s, sex in the 60s and 70s is often better for the woman than the man. At times, sex is one-way, although usually sexuality is mutual. After an accident or illness, sex energizes you emotionally and physically. When sex flows from pleasure to eroticism to orgasm, it affirms regularity and vitality as an aging couple. Sometimes sex is for comfort and solace after visiting a terminally ill sibling. A playful sexual encounter before a nap takes advantage of the flexibility of retirement. As couples age they are more likely to utilize self-entrancement arousal/eroticism. This is engaging for the giving partner and invites the receiving partner to bask in pleasure. GES enhances satisfaction at all ages. GES celebrates both mutual, synchronous as well as asynchronous experiences.

Illness, Disability, and Satisfaction

The good news is no illness or disability stops you from being sexual. The challenge is to accept the "new normal" and adapt couple sexuality to physical, psychological, and relational realities. Whether the issue is cancer, a stroke, loss of a limb or physical function, arthritis or pain, cardiac or lung function, you deserve sexual pleasure in your life. Cooperate to share pleasure and eroticism. Embrace the "new normal" without apology or self-consciousness. The essence of being a sexual woman is not a perfect body or perfect health. It is accepting your body with the illness or disability as you enjoy giving and receiving pleasure-oriented touch. Sexuality usually involves orgasm, but orgasm is not the core of satisfaction. A good example of satisfaction is sex after prostate cancer surgery. The man learns to enjoy pleasuring and eroticism without a firm erection. He also learns that he doesn't need an erection to experience orgasm. After prostate surgery he has orgasms, but no longer ejaculates out of his penis—the ejaculate goes into his bladder. Accepting the new normal and sharing sexuality is affirming for the man and couple. His acceptance of your body, including changes in arousal and orgasm with aging, affirms your sexuality.

Whether physical changes are a side-effect of illness or a result of multiple medications, these are accepted and adapted to. Sexual rehabilitation is part of a comprehensive treatment program for illness or injury. Touch and sexuality reaffirms that the illness/disability is a part of you but does not define you or control your sexuality. Maintaining desire and satisfaction illustrates positive coping with illness and disability. This includes the couple scheduling a joint consultation with the internist, oncologist, surgeon, cardiologist, psychiatrist, endocrinologist, or rehabilitation specialist. A couple consultation brings out the most helpful role for the physician, in terms of providing bio-medical information and support in dealing with your illness or disability, so that it does not control your sexuality. Be a knowledgeable, active patient who continues to value intimacy and sexuality. Deal with the medical issue as a couple. Illness and disability is an opportunity to enhance relational and sexual cooperation and satisfaction.

Summary

Satisfaction is the second most important dimension in the desire/pleasure/eroticism/satisfaction mantra. Orgasm is an integral component for satisfaction, but satisfaction is much more than orgasm. Orgasm as an individual pass–fail performance goal subverts satisfaction. Satisfaction involves enhanced sexual self-esteem and feeling energizing and bonded as a couple.

Female orgasmic response is first class, not inferior to the stereotypic male orgasm pattern. Female orgasm is variable, flexible, complex, and individualistic. Few women follow the male model of a single orgasm during intercourse without additional stimulation. Even fewer women are orgasmic 100% of couple encounters. Your "orgasmic voice" is part of your erotic voice. It can involve orgasm with manual, oral, intercourse, rubbing, or vibrator stimulation. Orgasm can occur during the pleasuring phase, during intercourse, or in afterplay.

Accept your orgasmic voice (pattern) rather than feel pressure to achieve the "right" orgasm—multiple orgasms, "vaginal" orgasm, "G-spot" orgasm, hour-long orgasm, tantric orgasm, an emission during orgasm. Performance pressure results in secondary non-orgasmic response and low desire. Acceptance of your orgasmic voice as healthy is the foundation which allows you to add orgasmic feelings and sensations if you choose. Orgasm is the natural continuation of the pleasuring/eroticism process. There is not a "right" orgasmic response nor is orgasm an individual performance goal. Orgasm is a natural result of sharing pleasure and eroticism.

Satisfaction is much more than orgasm. Satisfaction affirms your sexual self-esteem and energizes your bond. Female orgasm is variable, flexible, complex, individualistic, and most important, first class. Your "orgasmic voice" affirms your sexuality. Afterplay enhances satisfaction whether you are orgasmic or not.

9

THE GOOD ENOUGH SEX (GES) MODEL

When couples stop being sexual, whether at 50, 60, or 70, it is almost always the man's choice. Traditional men stop being sexual in their 50s and 60s. "Wise" men can be sexual in their 60s, 70s, and 80s. Be his sexual ally and urge him to embrace the Good Enough Sex (GES) model which is the key to remaining a healthy sexual couple with aging.

Women find GES inviting and easy to accept because it is congruent with female sexual socialization and experience. The great majority of women learn sexuality as an interactive, variable, flexible experience. In contrast, the great majority of men learn sexuality as easy, highly predictable, and totally in their control. The adolescent male learns that sex response is autonomous—i.e. he gets spontaneous erections and goes to intercourse and orgasm with his first erection. He experiences desire, arousal, and orgasm without needing anything from his partner. Traditionally, the man is expected to have sex with "any woman, any time, any situation" with the demand for perfect performance.

Male sex was defined as individual performance with total control and predictability. This might work (even if not healthy) for men in their teens, 20s, and even 30s, but not for men in their 40s and older, especially not in married or partnered relationships. The truth is that the female model of intimate, interactive, variable, and flexible couple sexuality is superior to the male autonomous sex performance model (Foley, Kope, & Sugrue, 2012). Sadly, when men talk with peers they brag, lie, and one-up each other. Male peers do not affirm GES. Acceptance of GES is in the context of an intimate sexual relationship where you embrace GES for yourself and your relationship.

GES affirms that couple sexuality is inherently variable and flexible. The core of healthy sexuality is giving and receiving pleasure-oriented touching. Couple sexuality is a team sport not an individual pass–fail performance. The traditional performance approach demands predictable erection from the man and predictable orgasm (during intercourse) from the woman.

The best sex involves mutual, synchronous experiences where both partners are desirous, aroused, orgasmic, and satisfied. We are in favor of arousal, intercourse, and orgasm as well as mutual, synchronous sex. The great majority of sexual experiences are positive. However, even among happily married, sexually functional couples less than 50% of sexual encounters are synchronous. Couple sexuality is inherently variable—involving a range of motivations, roles, meanings, and outcomes. The sexual encounter can have a very different role and feeling for you than your partner. That is normal and acknowledges the complex roles and meanings of couple sexuality. For example, sometimes the man experiences the sexual encounter as a means to reconnect and feel a sense of attachment, while for you sex is driven by the desire for orgasm as a tension reducer. A sexual encounter later that week is better for him than you—for him sex is the celebration of a job promotion while you enjoy "going along for the ride." The next week, a sexual encounter results in his orgasm, but is not a satisfying experience, while you feel warmth and attachment even though you did not reach orgasm. These examples illustrate that GES is much more than sex function. GES involves roles, feelings, and meanings. Satisfaction involves feeling good about yourself as a sexual woman and bonded and energized as a sexual couple. Desire and satisfaction are more important than arousal and orgasm. This is a core understanding for the woman, man, and couple.

GES becomes even more important with the aging of the partners and relationship. The challenge is to embrace GES as genuine and first class. Ideally this would occur in younger years, although it is more likely to be adopted in your 40s or older.

A key for GES is acceptance that not all touching can or should proceed to intercourse. Perhaps 85% of sexual encounters will flow from pleasure to arousal to erotic flow to intercourse and orgasm. When the sexual scenario does not flow, you (or he) need not panic or apologize. There is nothing more anti-erotic than sexual self-consciousness and apologizing. Promote a seamless transition to an erotic, non-intercourse scenario or a sensual, cuddly scenario. Be aware that it is normal for 5–15% of sexual encounters to be dissatisfying or dysfunctional. GES reinforces positive, realistic sexual expectations. Romantic love beliefs and perfect sex performance expectations subvert sexual desire and satisfaction.

GES Experiences and Expectations for Women

Most, although certainly not all, adult women find the GES model inviting. The easiest concept to adopt is valuing sensual, playful, and erotic scenarios rather than all touching proceeding to intercourse. The great majority of women, including those who are not orgasmic during intercourse, enjoy intercourse. However, the demand that all sexual touch has to proceed to intercourse leads to sex being a mechanical routine rather than an anticipated pleasure. Valuing alternate scenarios and erotic unpredictability puts spice into your sexual life. Sensual scenarios are different than playful scenarios which in turn are different than erotic scenarios. Value sensuality, playfulness, eroticism, and unpredictability. Freedom to enjoy both synchronous and asynchronous sex is empowering. An example is enjoying pleasuring your partner to orgasm rather than having intercourse when you are not desirous of intercourse. Freedom to broaden your sexual repertoire builds anticipation and a sense of deserving. A particularly powerful scenario is requesting your partner orally stimulate you to orgasm (or multiple orgasms) without the demand that it be reciprocated. GES recognizes that not all sexual experiences need to be serious, mutual, or have the same meaning for both partners.

Positive, realistic expectations are particularly important in regard to intercourse. Couples find mutual, synchronous intercourse is most valuable and meaningful. However, you (or your partner) is free to say, "This won't be an intercourse night—can we cuddle, play erotically, or take a rain check?" This is acceptable as long as it is not manipulative, and you don't blame your partner or feel blamed. Celebrate sexual variability and flexibility. Even the 15% of women who are orgasmic only during intercourse welcome sensual and playful scenarios as well as manual, oral, or rubbing stimulation. Variable, flexible sensual and sexual scenarios are integral to female and couple sexuality.

GES Experiences and Expectations for Men

For men, adopting the GES approach is a major challenge. He needs your support and enthusiasm. Reading and talking about variable, flexible GES is necessary, but not sufficient. You need to experience a sensual, playful, or erotic scenario and the pleasure that comes from non-intercourse sexuality. He can learn to "piggy-back" his arousal on yours. Your involvement and enthusiasm is good for you and helps him embrace GES.

Carolyn and Ian

Ian and Carolyn had been a couple for six years. This was 44-year-old Ian's first marriage and 45-year-old Carolyn's second. One factor that attracted Carolyn was that Ian was a confident, involved lover. He was sensitive to Carolyn's emotional, touch, and sexual needs unlike the first husband who was a "meat and potatoes" sex man. The first husband's foreplay scenario involved breast and vaginal stimulation to get Carolyn ready for intercourse. He would push intercourse four—five times a week, and she would reluctantly go along once or twice a week. At first sex was functional, but after the first year Carolyn's desire was low. She viewed intercourse as a way to placate him with little pleasure for herself. The marriage ended eight months after their daughter was born because Carolyn felt the first husband was a disappointment as a person, spouse, and father. He further disappointed her by having marginal contact with the daughter and made infrequent child support payments.

In the three years before meeting Ian, Carolyn found a renewed sexual desire with the dating scene. She had two romantic love/passionate sex/idealized relationships, each lasting less than a year. The relationship with

Ian started in that manner, but with time intimacy grew rather than burning out. Carolyn was open to creating an intimate relationship with Ian.

At 38 Ian wanted more from life than a six-month—two-year relationship. Ian wanted a life partner. He had grown fond of Carolyn's daughter and felt that the daughter deserved love and stability in her life. Carolyn found this touching. It increased her attraction to Ian and desire for a respectful, trusting, intimate marital commitment.

Although most sexual touching did lead to intercourse, it was a very different experience for Carolyn than with the ex-husband. Ian enjoyed touching both outside and inside the bedroom and sensed her feelings and needs rather than pushing for intercourse as quickly as possible. Intimacy, touching, and sexuality truly had a 15–20% role in their relationship. With normal ups and downs, sexuality had an energizing, bonding role for 16 years which included Ian adopting the daughter.

Ian had his first experience with erectile difficulty when he was 41. It was clear to Carolyn that the cause was fatigue and alcohol. He tried twice more that night, but Carolyn lacked desire and Ian was frustrated with the erectile difficulties. The next night intercourse went fine, and Carolyn thought nothing more about the problem. In her life she had occasional experiences of low desire or arousal. Like many women, Carolyn wasn't aware of the negative impact of the erectile problem on Ian. He no longer felt confident and unselfconscious about sex. Although he enjoyed pleasuring and eroticism, Ian rushed intercourse because he feared losing his erection. Over time erectile anxiety increased, as did the number of unsuccessful intercourse attempts.

Carolyn and Ian did not speak directly about challenges to couple sexuality. Carolyn developed a pattern of manually stimulating Ian to orgasm if he wasn't aroused enough for intercourse. For a number of months this worked fine, but Carolyn began resenting Ian's "sexual selfishness" and noticed a further decline in her desire. She loved Ian, but sexuality was no longer fun or energizing. Ian's making sure Carolyn was orgasmic before attempting intromission had the paradoxical effect of increasing her orgasmic response but decreasing her sexual desire.

With the airways flooded by Viagra ads, Carolyn encouraged Ian to ask the internist for a prescription. The doctor was glad to do so, although he gave Ian no guidance about how to use the medication other than not to drink alcohol before taking Viagra. Pro-erection medications have two major effects. The first is to increase efficacy of the vascular system so that once aroused the erection is firm and lasting. The second is psychological—Viagra serves as a placebo to reduce anticipatory anxiety. For a period of months, the fun was back in their sexual relationship. Ian's sexual enthusiasm increased Carolyn's sexual desire. However, this came to a crashing halt the first night Viagra failed to produce an erection sufficient for intercourse. Ian lost his sexual confidence and returned to avoidance. Carolyn begged him to try again and offered to stimulate him to orgasm, but to no avail.

After four months of a total sexual shutdown, Carolyn insisted they make an appointment with a couple sex therapist. Ian literally had to be dragged to the session. Couple sex therapy is more effective than a stand-alone pro-erection medication (Rosen, Miner, & Wincze, 2014). Ian was relieved that the therapist was empathic and respectful rather than berate or shame him. The therapist was clear that regaining erectile comfort and confidence was a couple challenge, and Carolyn had a crucial role in the process. The most important thing the clinician said was that Viagra would not return Ian to the autonomous, totally predictable erections of his youth. The therapist introduced the GES approach and gave them a handout with guidelines to read and discuss (Metz & McCarthy, 2004). This helped Ian and Carolyn develop positive, realistic expectations for change, rather than hoping a "magic pill" would guarantee erections.

The next step was an individual session with each partner for a psychological/relational/sexual history. In her session, Carolyn had a chance to voice her confusion, anxiety, and anger about relational and sexual matters. The clinician was supportive and empathic, normalizing Carolyn's feelings as well as making clear her positive role in the change process. Carolyn valuing desire/pleasure/eroticism/satisfaction was a crucial factor in the success of sex therapy. She had an opportunity to ask questions and clarify feelings about sensual, playful, and erotic scenarios as well as what she enjoyed about intercourse. When sex did not flow, Ian and Carolyn could transition to an erotic or sensual scenario, so the sexual experience would end in a positive manner. The therapist encouraged Carolyn to value mutual erotic scenarios in addition to pleasuring

Ian to orgasm. Carolyn was hopeful this would be a new, satisfying chapter in their sexual relationship.

Ian's individual session allowed him to create a new narrative about his psychological, relational, and sexual strengths and vulnerabilities. Ian needed to give up the traditional male demand for totally predictable sex performance. Ian liked the concept of "beating the odds" and learning to value variable, flexible, pleasure-oriented GES. The therapist encouraged Ian to ask his internist for a prescription for Cialis. The daily low dose Cialis regimen was easy to integrate into their couple style of intimacy, pleasure, and eroticism (Weeks & Gambecia, 2000). In addition, it allowed freedom of when to initiate sex. Ian was strongly encouraged to accept GES as first-class male sexuality and cautioned against expecting 100% predictable erections. Turning toward Carolyn as his intimate sexual ally was integral to couple sex therapy. A major new learning for Ian was to "piggy-back" his arousal on hers.

In subsequent therapy sessions these learnings were discussed, modified, and implemented. Change is seldom easy or problem-free; it's "two steps forward, one step back." GES was easier for Carolyn to accept than Ian. Ian would have preferred a return to the predictable erections and intercourse of his 20s. Interestingly, Carolyn's desire was enhanced by the variety and unpredictability of sexual scenarios and intercourse experiences. Choice, freedom, and unpredictability enhance desire.

Ian preferred to transition to intercourse and orgasm on his first erection. The therapist affirmed this preference and added two suggestions. First, do not transition to intercourse until he was into an erotic flow and utilize multiple stimulation during intercourse to build erotic flow (7–8 subjective arousal) to orgasm. Second, practice transitioning to erotic or sensual scenarios so he didn't panic if the sex did not flow to intercourse. Ian was positive about the first suggestion, but ambivalent about the second. Carolyn's enthusiasm about alternate sensual and erotic scenarios won Ian over. Reading and talking about alternative scenarios is important, but the real learning comes with implementing and practicing these. Variable, flexible GES was good for Carolyn, Ian, and their relationship.

Female Sexual Self-Acceptance

Traditionally, the woman felt she had to catch up with her partner—his desire, spontaneous erection, and readiness for intercourse was faster. New scientific findings and clinical insights establish that female sexual desire and orgasm are first class, not inferior to male sexuality (McCarthy & Wald, 2016). Female sexual response is more complex, variable, flexible, and individualistic than male response—different, not better or worse. Acknowledging and embracing desire/pleasure/eroticism/satisfaction is empowering. A prime guideline is to own your sexual voice, including your orgasmic voice.

The GES model accepts female sexual desire and orgasm as healthy. Female sexual socialization and experiences reinforce the value of variable, flexible, pleasure-oriented GES. It confronts the traditional male individual perfect performance model. GES is compatible with your sexual experience. Women accept the core concept—couple sexuality is a variable, flexible, pleasure-oriented experience where you share intimacy and eroticism. Orgasm is not a pass–fail test for you (and erection is not a pass–fail test for him). Intercourse is valued as the natural continuation of the pleasuring/eroticism process, not a pass–fail test. Desire and satisfaction are more important than arousal and orgasm. Acceptance of your body, touching, and the process of sharing sexuality is more important than individual sex performance. GES empowers you to embrace healthy sexuality rather than feel intimidated by sex performance demands.

Psychologically, the challenge is to accept variable, flexible sexuality as first class for you and your relationship. Biologically, accept your body and adopt healthy behavioral habits of sleep, exercise, eating, moderate or no drinking, and no smoking. Relationally, turn toward your partner as your intimate sexual friend and ally. There is no need to prove anything to him, yourself, or anyone else. GES is first-class sexuality.

Male Sexual Self-Acceptance

Traditionally, male sexual self-acceptance was contingent on perfect performance. He was afraid of failing his partner, and even more afraid of male peers knowing about his sexual problems. That's a hard way to live. If his penis could speak it would say "Treat me better, I am always one failure from being rejected and shamed."

GES builds a new foundation for male sexual awareness and acceptance. GES affirms he and his penis are human, not a performance machine. GES emphasizes each person's right to sexual pleasure and to turn toward the partner as an intimate and erotic friend rather than someone to perform for. GES allows the man to be self-accepting rather than afraid or shameful. Unfortunately, he will not receive support for GES from male friends. He needs acceptance from you in order to embrace GES.

Why is GES so hard for men to accept? The male performance model is oppressive. Boys, adolescents, young adults, and adult men have over learned the message that a "real man is willing and able to have sex anytime, anywhere, with any woman." Is this healthy? The man is afraid to challenge this because he fears being labeled a "loser," "wimp," or "not man enough." GES is belittled as "settling" because he can't "perform like a real man."

This irrational thinking and peer pressure subverts sexual self-esteem. You can't do it for him but can urge him to embrace GES and build sexual self-acceptance as a healthy man in a first-class relationship. His challenge is to take the risk and be a wise man who values couple sexuality. Don't be a traditional man who falls into the trap of anticipatory anxiety, rushes to intercourse, and experiences frustration, embarrassment, and eventually sexual avoidance. A wise man values intimacy, pleasure, and eroticism; enjoys giving and receiving sensual and playful touch; is open to erotic scenarios and techniques; transitions to intercourse at high levels of erotic flow; enjoys giving and receiving multiple stimulation during intercourse; allows erotic sensations to naturally culminate in orgasm; and enjoys the afterplay experience. This is a more involving, multidimensional sexual scenario than he experienced in his 20s, which is all to the good.

When there is not erotic flow to intercourse rather than trying to force sex, he transitions to a mutual erotic scenario, pleasures you to orgasm with his mouth or hands, or asks you to pleasure him to orgasm. An alternative scenario is saying "Tonight won't be an intercourse night so let's enjoy a sensual, cuddly scenario and be sexual in the next couple of days." You can welcome and enjoy erotic and sensual scenarios as long as he is positive and involved. GES is empowering for the woman, man, and couple.

Use of Pro-Erection Medications, Penile Injections, and Testosterone

Healthy women, men, and couples use psychological, bio-medical, and relational resources to promote sexuality. Pro-erection medications, penile injections, and testosterone enhancement are compatible with GES. The reason medical interventions have not been as successful as advertised is that no one (doctor or therapist) sits with the couple (or the man alone) and discusses how to integrate the medical intervention into their couple sexual style of intimacy, pleasuring, and eroticism (Leiblum, 2002). The medication/marketing approach overpromises easy, predictable erections. The 85% guideline for intercourse proposed by GES is applicable to couples using Viagra or Cialis. Few men return to totally predictable erections.

When the man uses medical resources to improve sexual confidence and function what are the guidelines for the couple? The ideal guideline is that you meet as a couple with the internist, urologist, endocrinologist, psychiatrist, or sexual medicine specialist. The first physician to consult is the internist who will assess medical factors such as high blood pressure, cardiac problems, diabetes, side-effect of medications, or a pituitary tumor.

Many couples prefer Cialis to Viagra because it provides freedom of when to be sexual. The crucial factor is he needs to feel desire and subjective arousal before the positive vascular effects of the medication kick in.

A crucial psychosexual skill is to not rush to intercourse as soon as he's erect. The rush to intercourse is driven by fear of losing his erection. Fear motivation does not promote sexual pleasure or function. A better strategy is for you to take the lead in transitioning to intercourse when you feel he (as well as you) are into an erotic flow. Another technique is for you to guide intromission. Rather than being distracted by intercourse concerns, he enjoys giving and receiving erotic stimulation. Multiple stimulation during intercourse facilitates the erotic experience for both of you.

The more intrusive the medical intervention the more likely it will produce an erection. An example is penile injections. The reason injections have been disappointing for so many couples and have such a high dropout rate is that it feels mechanical. He has difficulty ejaculating because he is not subjectively aroused, and you don't enjoy intercourse because you're not aroused. The sexual experience does not feel genuine or satisfying. If he chooses to use penile injections, do so in a manner which enhances involvement and subjective arousal. Schedule a couple consultation with the urologist or internist. Both you and your partner learn to do the injections. Many men feel more comfortable with you administering the penile injection. What is your preference?

The medical intervention can't be expected to provide everything sexually. A crucial psychosexual skill is engaging in pleasuring/eroticism to enhance his (and your) subjective arousal rather than assume he is subjectively aroused because he has an erection. Remember, communicate how to integrate the medical intervention or medication into your couple sexual style of intimacy, pleasuring, and eroticism (Nobre, 2017). This is a couple challenge—the injection can't do it for you.

Testosterone enhancement is becoming popular for both men and women. Although testosterone is sold at drug stores and on the internet, we strongly advise you to consult a competent endocrinologist with a sub-specialty with hormonal factors in sexual function. The trend to misuse and overuse testosterone is worrisome (Fine, 2017). Testosterone is usually prescribed in gel form but can be administered through patch or injection. Very seldom is oral testosterone used. Testosterone is a resource to enhance sexual desire for women and men who experience significant testosterone deficit. In those cases, testosterone is necessary, but not sufficient. Psychological, relational, and psychosexual skill factors need to be addressed to promote sexual receptivity and responsivity. With the impetus of testosterone, the person finds it easier to reestablish sexual anticipation.

Exercise: Accepting and Implementing the GES Approach

This couple exercise asks you to read, discuss, and, most important, implement the GES approach. Very few couples begin their sexual relationship with awareness of GES. Commonly, they begin as a romantic love/passionate sex/idealized (limerance) couple. This is a very special phase providing wonderful memories. However, by its nature the limerance phase ends after 6–24 months. It needs to be replaced by a couple sexual style which promotes strong, resilient sexual desire. Ideally, you explore and adopt the GES approach in your 20s or 30s. However, most couples do not do this until there are sexual problems, most commonly erectile dysfunction. Prevention is always superior, but the majority of couples do not adopt GES until a problem occurs. The good news is it's never too late to adopt GES. That is a wise decision for the woman, man, and couple.

Knowledge is power, so reading about GES is worthwhile. Even more important is a couple dialogue about the role and meaning of GES. The best time to talk about sexual issues is the day before being sexual, over a glass of wine or cup of tea, at the kitchen table or on the porch (clothed and sitting up) where you focus on sexual requests. The worst time to talk sex is in bed, nude, lying down, after a negative experience. The hurt, confusion, or anger causes people to say and do things which are harmful and destroy sexual confidence.

Genuine sexual communication involves sharing information/attitudes, making sexual requests, and, most important, disclosing sexual feelings. Don't be shy or give the socially desirable answer. Share both positive feelings as well as vulnerabilities. Be genuine and forthcoming about what you find positive and inviting about GES as well as any fears and concerns. Adopting GES is a couple challenge.

The suggested format to facilitate implementing GES involves practicing three sexual scenarios:

1. Transitioning to a mutual or asynchronous erotic scenario.
2. Transitioning to a sensual, cuddly scenario.

3. Practicing an intimate, interactive scenario which promotes intercourse as a natural continuation of the pleasuring/eroticism process. Transition to intercourse at high levels of erotic flow and utilize multiple stimulation during intercourse.

Most couples (especially men) prefer the intercourse scenario. This is fine as long as it is not a performance mandate or the only acceptable option.

We suggest practicing each scenario at least twice, and preferably three times. Hopefully, you become comfortable and confident with all three scenarios. A variable, flexible sexual repertoire is a great relational resource, especially in your 60s, 70s, and 80s.

Some couples decide not to incorporate one scenario or part of a scenario. For example, they say "Let's take a rain check" rather than engage in a sensual scenario. Some women prefer pleasuring their partner to orgasm rather than engaging in a mutual erotic scenario. Be honest with yourself and your partner about feelings and preferences as well as what does not fit. You are free to repeat parts of this exercise in the future—reading, talking, and implementing scenarios.

Guidelines for Asynchronous Sexual Scenarios

Couples prefer mutual, synchronous scenarios involving intercourse and orgasm. In addition, couples who enjoy asynchronous scenarios (both intercourse and erotic experiences) have a valuable GES resource.

A crucial guideline is that the asynchronous scenario cannot be at the expense of the partner or the relationship. Said positively, the scenario is a "3" or "6" on the pleasure scale for the less-involved partner. At a minimum, the asynchronous scenario is neutral. If it's negative, resentment grows and desire wanes.

A traditional example is the man enjoys intercourse and is orgasmic while you find it pleasant—whether a "4" or a "7." Often for couples over 60, female arousal and orgasm is easier than for the man. The erotic scenario where he pleasures you to orgasm is a "10" for you—the experience might be a "2" or "8" for him—he may or may not be orgasmic.

Another example is the man finds rear entry intercourse highly erotic, where you find it a "2" or "5." A further example is where you find a combination of oral vulva stimulation and manual anal stimulation to multi-orgasmic response highly satisfying, where he finds it a "3" or "6."

When there is a conflict over sexual scenarios we suggest couple sex therapy (Appendix A has guidelines for choosing a competent therapist). Sexual power struggles are destructive for the woman, man, and couple. You lose track of the goal of sharing pleasure; the agenda is not being the loser in the power struggle. Some couples decide not to engage in asynchronous scenarios. The majority of couples value asynchronous sexuality which acknowledges variable, flexible sexual response. Obviously, GES is compatible with asynchronous sexuality.

Summary

GES validates the reality of your sexual relationship. Flexible couple sexuality reinforces that the essence of a sexual encounter is giving and receiving pleasure-oriented touching. GES recognizes the multiple roles, meanings, and outcomes of sexuality for the woman, man, and couple. Intercourse and orgasm is highly valued, but not as an individual performance demand. Sexuality is much more than intercourse and satisfaction is much more than orgasm. Touching (affection, sensual, playful, erotic) is valued both inside and outside the bedroom—not all touch leads to intercourse. GES is of value to both partners. Your acceptance and enthusiasm for GES is crucial for your partner. GES especially thrives as an intimate team experience with aging.

Wise men accept GES. It helps the man rid himself of the oppressive male pass–fail performance test of erection and intercourse.

GES empowers the woman, man, and couple to accept variable, flexible sexuality with its multiple roles, meanings, and outcomes.

Approximately 85% of sexual encounters involve pleasure, arousal, erotic flow, intercourse, and orgasm. When the sexual encounter does not flow to intercourse, you transition to an alternative erotic or sensual scenario. Although the GES approach is more of a challenge for the man, it facilitates female, male, and couple sexuality into your 60s, 70s, and 80s.

10

DEVELOPING YOUR COUPLE SEXUAL STYLE

Two major contributions that the sex therapy field brings to couple relationships are utilizing psychosexual skill exercises to enhance sexual comfort and confidence and the value of developing a couple sexual style (which is often different than your relational style).

There are two components of your couple sexual style. First, maintain your sexual autonomy ("sexual voice") while being an intimate sexual team. Second, how you integrate intimacy and eroticism into your relationship. This is different than the relational style which focuses on how couples deal with practical and emotional differences and conflicts.

The primary couple sexual styles (by frequency) are:

1. Complementary (mine and ours).
2. Traditional (conflict minimizing).
3. Best Friend (soul mate).
4. Emotionally Expressive (fun and erotic).

Each couple sexual style has strengths and each has vulnerabilities (traps). Adopt a sexual style that meets her, his, and our needs and preferences. Reach a mutual agreement on which sexual style is the best fit. Your couple sexual style is then modified so that it meets your unique preferences (McCarthy & McCarthy, 2009).

A common self-defeating power struggle is the man wants the Traditional sexual style and you want the Best Friend style. This results in a chronic struggle, rather than sexuality being bonding for the couple. The

Complementary sexual style is the choice for the majority of couples, but not all. It is crucial that you reach a mutual emotional commitment of what you value about intimacy and sexuality. Remember, sexually one size never fits all.

We describe each couple sexual style focusing first on strengths, then vulnerabilities. Choose the couple style which is the best fit for your feelings, preferences, and values. Enjoy the strengths of your chosen style while monitoring traps so they don't subvert your sexuality.

Complementary Couple Sexual Style

The reason Complementary is the most common sexual style is that it fits the therapeutic model of each person being responsible for her sexuality while being an intimate sexual team. Both partners value intimacy and eroticism. In addition, you have "her," "his," and "our" bridges to sexual desire. Complementary couples are not sexual clones of each other. Each partner values intimacy, pleasuring, eroticism, intercourse, and afterplay. You affirm the value of both synchronous and asynchronous sexual scenarios. Acknowledge the multiple roles and meanings of sexuality including a shared pleasure, a means to reinforce intimate attachment, a tension reducer, and to conceive a planned, wanted child. In addition, sex affirms attraction, is a "port in the storm" when dealing with difficult parenting or financial issues, energizes your bond so you are motivated to resolve emotional conflicts, re-establishes a secure attachment, and provides comfort after a loss such as the death of a sibling (Metz, Epstein, & McCarthy, 2017). The Complementary style acknowledges the inherent variability and flexibility of couple sexuality. The Good Enough Sex (GES) approach is easily compatible with the Complementary couple sexual style.

The Complementary sexual style has a number of potential vulnerabilities. The major one is treating your sexual relationship with benign neglect, resulting in lowered desire and satisfaction even if sex remains functional. Another vulnerability is as life situations change (birth of a child, change of jobs) you don't incorporate that in your couple sexuality. The Complementary sexual style welcomes partner interaction and self-entrancement arousal scenarios. Role enactment arousal is more challenging to incorporate. Another potential vulnerability is you feel resentful that the promise of an equitable emotional and sexual relationship is not met.

Desire/pleasure/eroticism/satisfaction requires continued awareness and energy. You cannot treat your Complementary sexual style with benign neglect—sexuality cannot rest on its laurels.

Traditional Couple Sexual Style

This is the simple, stable, conflict minimizing sexual style. The couple adopt traditional gender roles—initiation is the man's domain with an emphasis on intercourse frequency. Intimacy and affection is your domain. There is little sexual fighting nor need for sexual negotiation—each partner is clear about their very different roles. Traditional sexual couples are usually religious, family-oriented, and enjoy community support. Same gender friends make jokes about the foibles of the opposite sex, but reinforce marital stability. Interestingly, this is the couple sexual style which more easily accepts a non-sexual relationship with aging, especially if you maintain an affectionate attachment.

There are several vulnerabilities of the Traditional sexual style. The most common is that sex roles become too rigid, causing isolation and alienation. The man believes you do not value intercourse. As he ages and deals with illness, including side-effects of medications, he has difficulty being sexually functional without your stimulation. Unfortunately, he turns away rather than toward you. The trap for you is resenting that his need for intercourse overrides your needs for intimacy and affectionate, including sensual and playful touch. You love your husband and feel loyal to the marriage, but no longer feel he is an intimate spouse nor do you value eroticism.

Another trap is dealing with infertility. Rather than seeing this as a medical issue where the couple needs to support each other, infertility is viewed as God's punishment for past sexual misdeeds. A further trap is that even though religious Catholics, Jews, Protestants, and Mormons are not supposed to have extra-marital affairs this occurs, including with happily married couples. The Traditional sexual couple finds it hard to recover from an affair (especially the woman's affair).

In dealing with difficult issues, we urge you to seek professional help and stay away from the traps of shame, blaming the spouse, or believing this is God's punishment for sex.

Best Friend Couple Sexual Style

Years ago when we wrote about couple sexuality, we said that the Best Friend sexual style was superior. That is what clinicians believed and since it was the couple sexual style that we adopted we thought it would be the best fit for others. How wrong we were. The Best Friend sexual style has strengths, but also great vulnerabilities. The Best Friend relational style is the best fit for the majority of couples, but not the Best Friend sexual style.

A major strength of the Best Friend sexual style is that you share intimacy and eroticism with the same person. Your partner knows your strengths and vulnerabilities and still loves and accepts you. If something goes wrong sexually, you trust he "has your back." The sense of mutuality, support, and the shared value of intimacy is very affirming.

Unfortunately, the Best Friend sexual style has major vulnerabilities. There is so much intimacy that you de-eroticize the partner. Also, mutuality is so crucial that you don't take personal and sexual risks. Asynchronous sexual experiences are difficult for Best Friend sexual couples to accept. This results in less sexual initiation and frequency. It is easier to be warm and cuddly than sexual and erotic. Best Friend couples have the most difficult time recovering from an extra-marital affair. They stay stuck, feeling betrayed by their best friend. Couples fall into the Best Friend sexual style because they mistakenly believe that if this style fits relationally it should fit sexually. The Complementary couple sexual style is a better fit for most couples.

Emotionally Expressive Couple Sexual Style

This is the fun and erotic sexual style. Other couples envy the Emotionally Expressive couple because they make their own rules, have lots of sexual energy, and have the most resilient sexual style. They bounce back from an extra-marital affair—they cry, yell, and have sex. They are open to a non-traditional life organization, enjoy role enactment arousal, and can have a consensual non-monogamy agreement.

The Emotionally Expressive sexual style has a large number of vulnerabilities, including that sexuality destabilizes your relationship. Even though resilient, after recovering from the fourth affair you feel emotionally worn out. The biggest vulnerability is breaking emotional and sexual boundaries. People are vulnerable sexually, especially when fighting about sex in bed, lying down, nude, after a negative sexual experience. When hurt, angry, or drunk, partners say harmful things that are long remembered. Examples include the man saying, "You pulled a sexual bait and switch—if I knew who you really were I never would have married you." Or the woman saying, "If you can't keep it up why do you bother to stay alive?" The partner apologizes the next day, but the put down does major harm to self-esteem and your relationship.

The guideline is play to the strengths of your chosen sexual style and be sure not to fall into the common traps. Your sexual style allows sexuality to play a 15–20% role in your relationship—energizing your bond and reinforcing feelings of desire and desirability.

Sarah and Mitch

When they married Sarah and Mitch were a loving, enthusiastic couple. After four years and one child it was unclear whether they would stay married. Rather than sexuality having a positive role, it had a 50–75% draining role, threatening marital stability.

Sarah and Mitch began as a romantic love/passionate sex/idealized couple. Sex was special and energizing. Sexual quality and frequency were excellent. This began changing after living together for five months. As they shared their lives and negotiated emotional and practical details including wedding planning, the "magic sex" phase ended. The issue was a common struggle—initiation patterns and intercourse frequency. Mitch pushed sex almost every day which caused Sarah to feel pressured. Sarah was pro-sexual and hated being stuck in the traditional female role of the sexual gatekeeper. She hoped this would improve after the wedding, but instead it intensified. Was it Mitch's fault, Sarah's fault, or was there something wrong with them as a couple?

Sarah looked forward to the honeymoon in Hawaii. Sadly, the honeymoon made the intercourse frequency problem worse. They argued every day. The two times they had intercourse it was functional for Mitch, but not Sarah, and both felt disappointed.

Sex with the goal of becoming pregnant was fun, but the pattern of conflict over intercourse frequency continued throughout the pregnancy and became worse after the baby was born. Mitch and Sarah enjoyed parenting and shared much in their lives, but were not an intimate sexual team.

Over the past eight months, Sarah was thinking seriously about divorce. Mitch did not want a divorce, but was tired of masturbation being his sexual outlet (in the past year they'd had intercourse three or four times; there was no sensual, playful, or erotic touch). Sarah no longer felt sexual desire with Mitch, but was increasingly attracted to other men.

Sarah's sister did an extensive internet search and found a respected pro-marriage sex therapist. The therapist was willing to see Mitch and Sarah for an initial couple session.

At the first session, it was clear that Sarah and Mitch were a demoralized couple who were caught in the blame—counter-blame cycle. This is typical for couples in a non-sexual marriage.

The clinician was not discouraged. She empathized about how demoralizing it was to go from being a loving, sexually vibrant couple to a non-sexual, alienated couple. She recommended they commit to a six-month therapy contract with the goal of creating a marital bond of respect, trust, and commitment and developing a new couple sexual style. Sarah was motivated by the therapist's willingness to work with them and especially struck by the therapist's optimism that like three out of four couples, Sarah and Mitch could develop a couple sexual style with revitalized desire. Mitch was hopeful because the clinician was experienced and suggested positive, realistic goals rather than promising a return to the magical sex of the first year.

Couple sex therapy requires focus and energy from both the couple and clinician. There are five clients (dimensions) for the therapist to attend to: 1. Sarah, 2. Mitch, 3. their relationship, 4. their sexual relationship, and 5. the most difficult client—their emotional and sexual history.

A major challenge in working with Mitch was his anger at Sarah for unfairly blaming him for the sexual problem. The clinician noted that Mitch couldn't change the past, although he could learn from the past. Mitch needed to focus on the present and future and accept that the desire problem was the joint enemy. In her individual session, Sarah committed to focus on the marriage rather than allow herself to be diverted by an affair—including an emotional, unconsummated affair.

The challenge for Sarah was to revive her sexual voice and rebuild positive anticipation—the core of sexual desire. An empowering psychosexual skill exercise gave Sarah the power to veto a sexual scenario. Mitch would honor her veto and stay involved rather than go away and sulk. Sarah and Mitch developed a trust position where she put her head on his heart, he stroked her hair, and they were mindful of feeling safe and attached. This was a powerful healing experience for Sarah.

You do not have the freedom to say "yes" to sex unless you have the power to say "no" and trust your partner will respect your veto. Your emotional needs are more important than his sexual wants. Rather than turning away, Mitch and Sarah turned toward each other in a sensual or sexual manner.

Mitch read material about couple sexual styles, took a questionnaire, and discussed their sexual attitudes, experiences, feelings, and preferences. In retrospect they understood the conflict—Mitch assumed they would have a Traditional sexual style and Sarah assumed they would have an Emotionally Expressive sexual style. This difference in assumptions and understandings guaranteed a sexual power struggle. The struggle about sex frequency had not been caused by negative motivation. They committed to revitalizing sexual desire as an intimate sexual team.

Sarah and Mitch (with the therapist's guidance) approached the choice of sexual style from a positive knowledge base with the assumption that both wanted a sexual style which was the best fit for them. The majority of couples in therapy choose the Complementary couple sexual style.

Sarah valued intimacy and eroticism and realized how important her sexual voice was. Mitch committed to intimacy and nondemand pleasuring. He was open to Sarah's preferences for sensual, playful, erotic, and intercourse scenarios. They developed afterplay scenarios which increased emotional and sexual satisfaction even when the sexual encounter was mediocre or unsatisfying.

Mitch and Sarah embraced the Complementary couple sexual style and integrated that with the Best Friend relational style. This provided a solid foundation for a respectful, trusting, intimate commitment. They welcomed a planned, wanted second child. Sex with the goal of pregnancy is an aphrodisiac.

Rather than taking their marital bond and couple sexuality for granted, Sarah and Mitch committed to a relapse prevention program. They would attend six-month check-in sessions for two years to be sure changes were maintained and generalized. In addition, they set a new sexual growth goal for the next six months. If the relationship ran into trouble they would schedule a "booster session." They had come too far psychologically, relationally, and sexually to allow a relapse.

Couple Discrepancies in Desire

You are not clones of each other, especially not sexually. There are differences in what you value about intimacy, touching, and sexuality. Contrary to popular belief, these are not governed by gender stereotypes. Men in partnered relationships value intimate sexuality and women value erotic sexuality.

Your attitudes, behaviors, emotions, and values are more important than gender stereotypes. Be clear and specific about sexual scenarios and feelings that promote sexual desire for you.

An important guideline is to not fall into the pursuer—distancer trap. Sexual power struggles are in no one's interest. The typical struggle is intercourse or nothing. One of the reasons American couples have intercourse only a bit more than once a week is that they only have two dimensions (gears)—affection and intercourse. This negates the value of sensual, playful, and erotic touch for itself as well as a bridge to intercourse.

Focus on sexuality as an intimate team experience of sharing pleasure. Discussing the value of touch and attachment facilitates openness to affectionate, sensual, playful, and erotic touch in addition to intercourse. Touch is an invitation to connection rather than a demand for sex. An empowering guideline is to enjoy touch both inside and outside the bedroom without the expectation that all touch should lead to intercourse. Many women dread the man's erection because the erect penis is perceived as a demand for intercourse or at least his needing an orgasm. Welcome his erection as a sign of pleasure rather than a sexual demand.

Sexual desire is enhanced by freedom, choice, and unpredictability. Implementing this is easiest for the Complementary sexual style. The man finds they have more intercourse because this guideline allows the woman freedom to enjoy intimacy and touching rather than being afraid of turning him on unless she wants intercourse. The key for the Emotionally Expressive couple sexual style is to emphasize playfulness, unpredictability, and eroticism. The Traditional sexual style couples depend on the man to initiate sex. The Best Friend sexual style couple needs to be explicit about the behavioral cues which promote desire for intercourse.

Exercise: Discovering Your Couple Sexual Style

Choosing the right couple sexual style is a very important emotional decision which affects your relationship and sexuality for years. It is crucial to be honest with yourself and your partner. Discuss the following questions:

1. How important is sex in your life? How important is a satisfying, secure, and sexual relationship?

2. What is your preferred way to express affection—holding hands, kissing, or hugging?
3. For you, what is the difference between affectionate touch and sexual touch?
4. How much do you value sensual, non-genital touch? Do you prefer taking turns or mutually giving and receiving?
5. What is the meaning and value of genital pleasuring? Do you experience this as playful or is it always oriented toward intercourse? What is your favorite playful scenario? Do you enjoy mixing non-genital and genital touch?
6. Do you value erotic scenarios and techniques that do not lead to intercourse? Do you prefer manual, oral, rubbing, or vibrator stimulation? Do you enjoy multiple stimulation or do you prefer a single, focused stimulation? Taking turns or mutual stimulation? Using external stimuli (sex toys, erotic videos, playing out a fantasy)? Do you enjoy erotic sex to orgasm or as a prelude to intercourse?
7. Do you view intercourse as a natural extension of the pleasuring/eroticism process or a pass–fail sex performance test? Do you transition to intercourse as soon as possible or transition to intercourse at a high level of erotic flow? What is your preferred intercourse position? What type of thrusting do you most enjoy? Do you value multiple stimulation during intercourse?
8. How much do you value afterplay? What afterplay scenarios and techniques enhance satisfaction?
9. What is the preferred balance of your sexual voice (autonomy) with being an intimate sexual team?
10. How do you integrate intimacy (closeness, loving feelings, warmth, security, predictability) with eroticism (creativity, mystery, taking emotional and sexual risks, intense feelings and sensations, unpredictability)?

Discuss your feelings and preferences. Where are areas of agreement? Disagreement? To develop a comfortable, pleasurable, erotic, and satisfying couple sexual style you need to take personal responsibility and be committed to sharing intimacy, pleasuring, and eroticism.

Among the four couple sexual styles—Complementary, Traditional, Best Friend, and Emotionally Expressive—choose the style which affirms your sexual voice and allows you to be intimate and erotic allies.

Each partner states the one or two couple sexual styles which would be a good fit as well as one or two which would not be right for you. This is not an analytic problem-solving process, but an attitudinal/behavioral/emotional commitment of who you are as a sexual person and an intimate sexual team.

Ideally, both partners choose the same couple sexual style. When there is not agreement, engage in an emotional exploration of the couple sexual style each of you prefer. Do not fall into the demand/coerce mode. Share with your partner the key dimensions of your sexual voice, what you value about being an intimate sexual team, and your preferred way to integrate intimacy and eroticism. Listen empathically and respectfully to your partner's emotional and sexual preferences. This process increases understanding, empathy, and acceptance. A healthy intimate relationship is based on a positive influence process, with a commitment to not becoming stuck in a power struggle. One strategy is to spend one month playing out one sexual style and the next month playing out an alternative sexual style. Which sexual style best fits your needs? Find a genuine common ground where individually and as a couple your sexual relationship has a 15–20% role in energizing your bond. Once you have chosen your couple sexual style, individualize components so sexuality uniquely fits you.

Monitoring the Vulnerabilities of Your Chosen Couple Sexual Style

Each couple sexual style has its vulnerabilities (traps). Be aware so you don't fall into these. Individually and as a couple commit to taking action to address vulnerabilities. An advantage of choosing a couple sexual style is you don't have to monitor all the traps, only the ones relevant for your sexual style.

The Complementary couple sexual style has many strengths which is why it's the most chosen. The biggest vulnerability (trap) is complacency—you take sexuality for granted. Rather than devoting thought, energy, and communication so your Complementary sexual style remains vital and satisfying, sex becomes routine and stale. To address this vulnerability, we suggest each partner should introduce a new initiation scenario, a new pleasuring lotion or sequence, a new erotic scenario or technique, a new pattern of multiple stimulation during intercourse, a new intercourse position or thrusting rhythm, or a new afterplay scenario. Each partner initiates at least one new thing each year (a minimum of two new sexual scenarios a year). This ensures couple sexuality remains vital and satisfying.

The prime vulnerability for the Traditional couple sexual style is that the roles become rigid. As the man ages and his ability to function autonomously is limited, he becomes self-conscious and anxious. The trap for the woman is she resents that her needs for intimacy and touch are overridden by his need for intercourse and orgasm. The suggested intervention is once every six months he initiates an intimacy date with a prohibition on intercourse and orgasm. Every six months she initiates a playful or erotic scenario and it's her choice whether to transition to intercourse (less than 50% of the time she chooses to include intercourse). Honor traditional roles while "spicing up" your relationship.

The Best Friend couple sexual style's major vulnerability is with so much emphasis on intimacy you "de-eroticize" your partner. A second vulnerability is with so much emphasis on mutuality you take few personal or sexual initiations resulting in decreased sexual frequency. The suggested intervention is that once every six months each partner initiates a "selfish," asynchronous erotic scenario. Own your sexual feelings—it is normal and healthy to have different sexual preferences than your partner. This confronts the "tyranny of mutuality." It allows you freedom (as long as it's not at the expense of the partner or the relationship) to enjoy your sexual voice. Another intervention is to initiate a playful scenario—not all sex needs to be intimate and serious. Playfulness is a sign of healthy couple sexuality.

The vulnerability of the Emotionally Expressive couple sexual style is you wear each other out with emotional and sexual drama. When hurt or angry, the partner drops a "sexual atomic bomb." The intervention is to establish boundaries. Each partner highlights one—three sexually destructive issues. You agree that no matter how hurt, angry, or drunk you are, you will not launch a sexual attack. A specific suggestion is to not talk sex when lying in bed, nude, after a negative sexual experience. In that situation, people say and do things which can cause great damage.

Enjoy the strengths of your couple sexual style and monitor the traps so these do not subvert sexuality.

Gender Issues and Couple Sexual Style

The traditional simplistic belief that women value intimacy and men value intercourse has done great damage to women, men, couples, and the culture. The core concept behind choosing a couple sexual style is to have both partners speak the same intimacy and sexuality language. Each partner has her/his sexual voice and values being an intimate sexual team. Determine the right integration of intimacy and eroticism for you. The Traditional couple sexual style is organized along traditional gender roles, but affirms the importance of being a couple. The Complementary couple sexual style affirms female—male sexual equity, and gives each partner the right to initiate, say no, and value both intimacy and eroticism. A key element of the Complementary sexual style is to disarm the traditional male—female power struggle over intercourse frequency. The Best Friend sexual style emphasizes intimacy and mutuality. The Emotionally Expressive sexual style emphasizes both partners enjoying eroticism and taking sexual risks. The issue is which sexual style fits your feelings about gender roles and sexuality.

Summary

A major contribution the sexuality field brings to the relationship field is the importance of developing a couple sexual style which promotes and maintains sexual desire. There is not "one right" way to be a sexual couple, but it is crucial to choose the sexual style which is the best fit for you. Break the cycle of sexual power struggles. More important, promote desire/pleasure/eroticism/satisfaction.

Play to the strengths of your chosen sexual style and be aware of the vulnerabilities so you don't fall into these traps. Individualize your sexual style so it uniquely fits your feelings and preferences. Be sure your style allows sexuality to have a 15–20% positive role in your life and relationship.

Maintain your sexual voice while being intimate and erotic allies. Your couple sexual style is often different than your relational style. Your couple sexual style promotes sexual satisfaction and facilitates feelings of desire and desirability.

11

WOMEN AND MEN AS INTIMATE AND EROTIC ALLIES

Traditionally, men and women were assumed to be very different sexually. Men were assumed to have higher desire, be better sex performers, benefit from higher testosterone, and emphasize eroticism. Women lacked desire, had a difficult time reaching orgasm, less testosterone, and valued intimacy—not eroticism. In the 1980s the culture was seduced by the "pop psych" book "Men are from Mars, Women are from Venus." Simple and clear, but scientifically almost totally wrong (Hyde, 2005).

For adult women and men, especially in a married or partnered relationship, there are many more psychological, relational, and sexual similarities than differences. In fact, a study of couples married over 20 years conducted in five countries found that what women most valued in their long-term marriage/life partnership was a vital sexual relationship where she felt desire and desirable. What men most valued was a high degree of affection and security. In other words, the reverse of traditional male—female sexual assumptions (Heiman, et al., 2011).

The challenge for married/partnered couples is to integrate intimacy and eroticism to create strong, resilient desire. This is easier when both partners value intimacy and eroticism rather than the traditional gender split. Integrate your "erotic voice" into couple sexuality. Eroticism is core to female sexuality as it is to male sexuality. Males learn to value intimacy as core to male and couple sexuality.

Problematic issues with eroticism are the porn definition of what eroticism is and emphasis on role enactment scenarios. The performance-oriented anti-intimacy approach to eroticism is rigid and self-defeating. The healthy approach to eroticism emphasizes its integral role in the desire/pleasure/eroticism/satisfaction mantra. Integrated eroticism emphasizes partner interaction and self-entrancement arousal. Eroticism involves high levels of sensations and feelings (6–10 subjective arousal) which includes intercourse and orgasm, but is much more. The key is finding your "erotic voice." This provides you freedom to experiment with personally engaging sexual scenarios and techniques. Reject the porn model and belief that the man has power to approve or disapprove your erotic voice. You have a right to your erotic voice in the same way he has a right to his "intimate voice." Don't try to be clones of each other.

What scenarios and techniques allow you to experience intense emotional and sexual feelings? Is your preference partner interaction arousal, self-entrancement arousal, or role enactment arousal? Do not be "politically correct." What is the right fit for your erotic voice?

The most common pattern is partner interaction arousal/eroticism. However, it's not right if it doesn't fit for you. Most women find role enactment arousal intimidating rather than a turn-on. The question is what fits your feelings and preferences. Your partner has the right to veto scenarios and techniques that are aversive or intimidating for him. However, he does not have the right to avoid or take an anti-erotic stance. Both partners are actively involved and value erotic feelings and scenarios.

Traps to Avoid

The most common trap is overpromising and then feeling like a sexual failure. It is easy to say "we want to be intimate and erotic allies." Your challenge is to change attitudes, behaviors, and emotions to create a healthy sexual relationship. You don't need to be perfect nor do you need to be intimate and erotic allies every time. Couple sexuality is variable and flexible. By its nature couple sexuality is anti-perfectionistic.

A common trap is the rigid gender assumption that all women always value intimacy and that all men always value eroticism. Clarity is good, but rigidity subverts your sexuality. There are women who highly value eroticism and men who highly value intimacy. This changes over time and in different situations. For example, in recovering from surgery you seek sexual validation for the "new normal" of your body sexual function and image. Men can seek support and security in their relationship especially when dealing with parental or career disappointments. People are human first, including recognizing that intimacy and eroticism is important for personal well-being and a satisfying relationship.

Being intimate and erotic allies is crucial for a satisfying, secure, and sexual marriage (or life partnership). A common trap is to split intimacy and eroticism. Clinicians tire of hearing "I love my spouse, but I'm not in love with him." You value the relationship and family, but have lost sexual desire because you have de-eroticized him (and he has de-eroticized you). There is so much emphasis on closeness and mutuality that there is no space for playfulness and eroticism. Couples usually begin their relationship with a romantic love/passionate sex charge (limerance phase) which powerfully drives desire. However, the limerance phase is fragile, lasting six months to two years. The challenge is to develop a couple sexual style which integrates intimacy and eroticism. Sadly, that challenge is ignored and you fall into a sexual routine which may be functional, but does not energize your bond nor reinforce feelings of desire and desirability. The trap is not valuing erotic scenarios and techniques; sexuality loses its special charge. Your relationship falls into a dichotomy of intercourse or nothing, with nothing being the likely outcome (Brotto & Luria, 2014).

Contrary to media and "common sense" beliefs, problems with eroticism are as likely to occur with men as women. The trap for the man is associating eroticism with an illicit relationship or with the porn model of crazy, lustful performance. He does not value eroticism in an intimate relationship. The man splits and compartmentalizes eroticism. He ignores the desire/pleasure/eroticism/satisfaction mantra. A male trap is compulsively using on-line porn and negating the value of intimate, interactive couple sexuality to promote eroticism (Reid & Jorgensen, 2017).

The common trap for women is to negate your "erotic voice." You view eroticism as the man's domain and associate eroticism with porn or out of control male sexuality.

An extreme trap is placing so much value on intimacy that sexual playfulness and vitality is lost. This does not necessarily follow traditional gender stereotypes. There are males who put such emphasis on an intimate, cuddly, secure relationship that erotic feelings are perceived as anti-intimate. He loses sexual drive, erotic fantasies, and de-eroticizes his partner in the name of intimacy. The female trap is to become too comfortable with affection and closeness, and shut out erotic feelings and sensations. A loss for you and your relationship.

Value Being Intimate and Erotic Friends

Being intimate and erotic friends is a cognitive-behavioral-emotional commitment to a sexually satisfying relationship (Metz & McCarthy, 2010). Embracing both intimacy and eroticism halts the traditional gender wars and contingent approach to sexuality. Emotional and behavioral integration is the answer to the trap of "politically correct" slogans which disintegrate under challenges and stresses. Genuine intimacy means being a sexually healthy woman and accepting your partner for who he really is with strengths and vulnerabilities. Integrated eroticism is shared as part of desire/pleasure/eroticism/satisfaction. Accept eroticism as valuable for itself and not contingent on everything being perfect. Traditionally, women weren't supposed to feel erotic unless you felt secure and loved. Although we are strong supporters of secure and loving feelings, eroticism is healthier when it's not contingent. Eroticism is not contingent on everything being in emotional synchrony. Remember, integrated eroticism is not at the expense of the partner or relationship. Eroticism is valued with a range of roles, meanings, and outcomes (Perel, 2006).

Being intimate and erotic allies is an ongoing, dependable part of a healthy sexual relationship. Even when there is frustration, disappointment, or anger you do not stop being an intimate sexual team. You deal with problems as allies, not threaten to withdraw intimacy or sexuality. Deal directly with emotional and sexual problems; ignoring or avoiding results in problems becoming chronic and severe. Deal with issues as intimate and erotic allies; the likelihood of success is much better. The words that make a difficult situation unmanageable are "If you loved me you would." Another dramatic, self-defeating strategy is to stop being sexual until the emotional problem is resolved. The outcome is an increase in power struggles which makes it harder to dialogue and problem-solve. You become stuck in a non-sexual relationship where there is little or no touching.

Being intimate and erotic friends is important in both good and bad times, but especially during bad times. Knowing your partner "has your back" even when disappointed and angry is a powerful relational resource. Just as important is to maintain affectionate, sensual, playful, and especially erotic touch (which includes intercourse but is not limited to intercourse). This energizes you to deal with difficult emotional issues. Eroticism and sexuality play a number of roles from healing to energizing, and from intense emotion to tension reduction. Eroticism reenergizes you and reinforces feelings of desirability. Be aware that it is normal for the man to crave intimacy as a way to deal with sadness and hurt. Don't fall into traditional gender traps or allow yourself or your partner to split intimacy and eroticism. Turn toward your partner to promote couple sexual health.

Shauna and Royal

When they met eight years ago, Shauna and Royal were cynical about the opposite gender, the dating game, and sexuality. Royal's older brother had married at 21, and 29-year-old Royal sometimes wished he'd chosen the early marriage route. Royal was used to the up and down pattern of dating/sexual relationships, the erotic charge and optimism of a new love affair, and the disappointment, pain, and blaming when the relationship ended. Royal felt more emotionally and sexually sophisticated than at 21, but also more cynical about women and relationships.

Shauna was 31 when she met Royal. Her dating/sexual experiences were similar to his with the addition of two STIs and an abortion. Shauna accepted her psychological, relational, and sexual history with its strengths and vulnerabilities. There are things she regretted, but she did not feel shameful. Shauna processed her experiences with a female friend, a therapist, and after being a couple for a year with Royal.

Shauna wanted Royal as her emotional and sexual partner. She experienced him as a "good guy" who was low-key and non-judgmental. She respected and trusted Royal, believing he cared about her emotional and sexual feelings. After eight months of dating they began a serious dialogue about being intimate life partners, including marriage and children. Shauna knew she wasn't perfect and didn't expect Royal to be perfect. They talked about values and what it would mean to be a committed couple.

Shauna and Royal cohabitated for seven months before the wedding. Shauna approached living together as a trial period. If they could not share their lives she would not "slide" into marriage—she was committed to a satisfying, secure marriage and children.

Shauna and Royal have been married seven years with a 5-year-old daughter and a 3-year-old son. Shauna was glad they waited a year after marriage before becoming pregnant. Like most women, Shauna found the first two years of marriage challenging and hard work. They established a two-career lifestyle and a Best Friend marital style. Some life tasks were divided by traditional gender roles (Shauna was a better cook than Royal, although he did the cleanup and grocery shopping). Other tasks were divided differently than traditional roles (Shauna handled investments and Royal household expenses and bill paying). Both were actively involved parents.

Shauna roughhoused with the children and Royal was a nurturing parent who gave baths, changed diapers, and was an affectionate father. They were committed to being sex educators for their children. Shauna's mother had not been a positive sex educator for her or her siblings.

Shauna and Royal were comfortable with the Best Friend relational style—it was the right fit for their marriage. Shauna assumed that their couple sexual style would mirror their relational style. Unfortunately, this resulted in low sex frequency because unless everything felt "right" they were not sexually playful nor did she initiate intercourse. Shauna experienced inhibited desire with Royal, not feeling sexually desirable. Although sex was more frequent on vacation, it wasn't special. Royal's complaints about intercourse frequency were a major turn-off for Shauna. She missed the special feelings of the limerance phase. She knew she couldn't go back to the romantic love/passionate sex, but wondered "Is this all there is?" Their sex was mediocre; not energizing.

One day Shauna arranged a babysitter and she and Royal went for a hike. When they reached the pinnacle of the hill, they found a rock to sit on. Shauna produced a half-bottle of wine from her backpack, poured two cups, and asked Royal whether he was satisfied with their lovemaking. When he tried to divert the conversation to the frequency problem, she assertively asked him to stay with the quality issue. Royal assured Shauna he found her attractive and was not looking for another partner, but he too was disappointed with the quality of their sexual relationship.

The core issue is that although they were intimate friends, they were not erotic allies. Shauna had de-eroticized Royal and their relationship while Royal focused on intercourse frequency at the expense of pleasure and eroticism. They needed to develop a couple sexual style which reinforced desire/pleasure/eroticism/satisfaction. Good intentions and good words were important, but not enough. They needed a behavioral and emotional commitment to develop a new couple sexual style. There was no need to put a prohibition on intercourse, but there was a need to revitalize intimacy, pleasuring, and eroticism. To combat the traditional gender split, Royal was in charge of intimacy scenarios and Shauna in charge of erotic scenarios.

Shauna had a strong preference for partner interaction arousal/eroticism as well as being open to self-entrancement arousal/eroticism. She consulted books and websites for suggestions to enhance eroticism, but was put off that the majority of suggested techniques involved role enactment arousal—watching X-rated videos and playing out sexual fantasies. Shauna was turned-off by these strategies. Frankly, she felt they were stupid. If it worked for other women and couples that was fine, but it was not the right fit for Shauna and Royal.

What appealed to Shauna was partner interaction arousal/eroticism that encouraged the "give to get" guideline. She enjoyed sex play to high levels of erotic flow before transitioning to intercourse. A highly erotic scenario was Shauna being orgasmic with manual and oral stimulation before intercourse, transitioning to intercourse when highly aroused, engaging in multiple stimulation during intercourse, enjoying erotic fantasies, and being orgasmic. Shauna's sexual responsivity provided an erotic charge for Royal. He did not demand that erotic scenario each time. He realized that quality couple sexuality was more important than intercourse frequency.

Shauna found it easier to be orgasmic during erotic sexuality. She accepted that Royal preferred orgasm during intercourse, although on occasion it was erotically fulfilling being fellated when Shauna did not want intercourse. The pattern of the woman being orgasmic before intercourse and the man during intercourse is very common (Heiman, 2007).

Perhaps the most important erotic learning was that each partner was easily, reliably aroused with self-entrancement arousal. This was particularly important for Royal who learned to value "easy erections" when pleasured by Shauna. So many of his friends used Viagra rather than turn toward the partner as his erotic ally.

Royal wanted Shauna to be his erotic as well as intimate friend. Feeling valued as a sexual woman was affirming. Royal initiated intimacy dates, including arranging for a babysitter and making reservations for dinner or a concert. They shared a genuine bond. Shauna no longer felt she and the marriage were taken for granted. Intimacy and sexuality require ongoing attention, time, and energy—it cannot be treated with benign neglect.

Shauna and Royal committed to be in the 30% of married couples who maintained an intimate and erotic relationship while parenting. Enjoying a vital sexual relationship and feeling they were an intimate sexual team was different than the limerance phase. It felt less dramatic, instead genuine and solid. Maintaining a genuine intimate and erotic connection throughout the marriage requires time and energy, but this was so much better than the marginal relationship they'd experienced during the past few years. Shauna and Royal were committed to being intimate and erotic allies and reinforcing desire/pleasure/eroticism/satisfaction.

Good Enough Sex (GES) and Being Intimate and Erotic Friends

The GES concept is motivating and empowering for real-life couples even though it doesn't have the "pizzazz" of dramatic sex. GES recognizes that by its nature couple sexuality is variable and flexible with a range of roles, meanings, and outcomes. GES is compatible with being intimate and erotic allies. You share exceptional experiences, special experiences, energizing experiences, good sex, better than average sex, routine sex, okay sex, mediocre sex, frustrating sex, dissatisfying sex, and dysfunctional sex. The key is to turn toward each other rather than blame or panic. A core strategy is an anti-avoidance approach to touching and sexuality. Even when intercourse is problematic or dysfunctional, don't cease sensual, playful, and erotic sexuality. You have a commitment to stay physically and emotionally connected. As sexual friends you confront the blaming/shaming trap so many couples fall into. It's fun to be intimate and erotic allies when sex is good. It's reassuring to remain intimate and erotic allies when sex is dissatisfying or dysfunctional. That does not mean settling for bad sex. It means being an intimate sexual team who dialogue and problem-solve sexual concerns.

A poisonous power struggle is one partner (regardless of gender) blames the other who denies or avoids. GES stops this power struggle by reminding each partner that sexuality is a team sport and they need to treat each other as intimate and erotic friends, not enemies. The partner experiencing sexual problems has confidence that "he has my back." He wants to be your intimate and erotic ally and share pleasure and satisfaction.

GES honors the reality that couple sexuality is variable and flexible, with a range of roles, meanings, and outcomes. Although the media and most couples value spontaneous sexual encounters, the reality for the great majority of couples is that most sexual experiences are planned or semi-planned which is as genuine as spontaneous sex (Gillespie, 2017).

Sex which is always perfect is a wonderful fantasy, but that is not the reality and would be boring. The variability and complexity of couple sexuality demonstrates the importance of being intimate and erotic allies who join to deal with problems. Unfortunately, "sex experts" emphasize individual sex performance at the expanse of intimate, erotic couple sexuality.

Proponents of intimacy put down eroticism and proponents of eroticism speak of the smothering effects of intimacy. In GES, both intimacy and eroticism are necessary and valued. The couple challenge is to find the balance of intimacy and eroticism which promotes strong, resilient desire.

GES helps couples deal with the vicissitudes of life, including the ups and downs of maintaining an intimate sexual attachment. Life, intimacy, and sexuality are complex and challenging. Through it all, maintaining your intimate and erotic friendship is a major marital resource.

Exercise: Reinforcing Your Intimate and Erotic Relationship

The value of psychosexual skill exercises is to make personal and concrete concepts and guidelines. This exercise asks you and your partner to put these concepts into practice.

Each partner takes a turn designing and playing out an exercise to integrate intimacy and eroticism into your relationship. Remember, you are not clones of each other nor is this a competition.

You take the first turn and then he designs his scenario. Rather than organizing in the traditional manner of being intimate first and then erotic, we suggest experimenting with either doing this in tandem or starting with erotic playfulness. Don't reinforce the traditional pattern of eroticism being contingent on feeling secure and intimate. Eroticism is a valuable component of your sexual voice. It doesn't need to be justified by feeling intimate before feeling erotic.

Do you prefer erotic play inside or outside the bedroom? Do you prefer partner interaction arousal/eroticism, self-entrancement arousal/eroticism, or role enactment arousal/eroticism? Design an erotic scenario which is inviting for you and enhances your intimate connection.

For many women, partner interaction arousal with a self-entrancement component provides the best fit. Rather than starting in the bedroom, after children are asleep (or out of the house), go to the guest room or family room and lock the door. Put on your favorite music or burn a candle to set a seductive milieu. Rather than lying down, begin the scenario standing up (if there were a mirror in the room you could do this scenario in front of it). Begin touching with clothes on or semi-clothed; allow the touching to be sexy and playful. Enjoy giving and receiving touch. Rather than the traditional progression from affectionate to pleasurable to playful to erotic touch, how does it feel to mix it up starting with playful or erotic touch?

Women find that unless their subjective arousal is at least a 4 or 5, focused genital stimulation is counter-productive. Using the "give to get" pleasuring guideline, what is your preferred mix of giving and receiving touch? When you move away from the traditional "foreplay" scenario, most women realize that being passive with the man stimulating you to get ready for intercourse is not erotically inviting. Giving and receiving sensual, playful, and erotic touch is inviting. This allows you to be actively involved in the pleasuring/eroticism process.

When subjective arousal is in the 5–6 range, many women enjoy switching to self-entrancement arousal. This involves being mindful of erotic sensations and feelings, allowing your body to be receptive to intense sexual feelings. Actively embrace erotic sensations rather than passively accepting stimulation. Allow yourself to be responsive and enjoy erotic flow. Use fantasies as a bridge to heightened erotic feelings. Some women enjoy erotic flow to orgasm with manual and/or oral stimulation while others prefer to transition to partner interaction arousal and intercourse. What is your preferred erotic scenario(s)? It may be similar to those used by others or totally different. This is true of your intimate scenario—it might be similar to his or dissimilar. Sexual desire is facilitated by freedom, choice, and unpredictability. This exercise makes that concept personal and concrete. Some women feel greatest erotic intensity with manual stimulation, others oral stimulation, others through intercourse (usually involving multiple stimulation during intercourse), others with rubbing stimulation, and others with vibrator stimulation. Be aware of alternative erotic patterns. Give yourself permission to enhance your erotic experience.

What is your preferred way to integrate eroticism and intimacy? For some women intimacy is integral to the entire sexual scenario while others embrace the freedom of erotic expression. You can utilize an afterplay scenario to end the encounter in an intimate, bonding manner. Both eroticism and intimacy are valued and need to be balanced and integrated, but not for every sexual encounter.

You might prefer an initial focus on intimacy. This is fine as long as you integrate erotic scenarios and techniques.

Be open to your partner's scenario. Accept it; don't judge it as better or worse than yours. You have the right to veto a scenario which is intimidating or a turn-off, but not the right to avoid. Be open to alternative intimacy/erotic scenarios.

Summary

Couple sexuality is complex and challenging with a range of roles, meanings, and outcomes. Commit to being intimate and erotic friends in both good and bad times, relationally and sexually. Intimacy and eroticism are very different dimensions, but not adversarial or incompatible. Intimacy builds loving, close, secure, predictable, and meaningful attachment. Eroticism builds a vital, vibrant, unpredictable, and emotionally and sexually charged relationship. Both the woman and man value intimacy and eroticism—not split by traditional gender roles. Value your erotic voice for yourself and your relationship. Your partner values intimacy for himself as well as the relationship.

Eroticism is not contingent on all aspects of the relationship being positive. Eroticism energizes you and is a couple resource for dealing with disappointments and frustrations.

Finding the balance of intimacy and eroticism is crucial; there is not one right integration which fits all women and all couples. Confidence that he is your intimate and erotic friend is crucial. This is a powerful resource against inhibited sexual desire. Knowing that your partner views you as his intimate and erotic ally reinforces that you are a sexual team committed to desire/pleasure/eroticism/satisfaction. Do not split intimacy and eroticism. The challenge is to integrate intimacy and eroticism as a woman and as a couple. You have a right to your erotic voice.

12

SATISFYING, SECURE, AND SEXUAL MARRIAGE

Women (and mental health professionals) were taught that marital satisfaction and security were a package. Love and communication were all that was necessary for a satisfying sexual relationship. These simplistic overpromises have led to disappointment and alienation (as well as a high divorce rate). You are disappointed with the man, the marriage, and sex. You conclude this is a "fatally flawed" marriage.

Throughout this book we advocate for your sexual voice as a healthy woman and for a relationship which is satisfying, secure, and sexual. These are three separate dimensions; do not assume they naturally go together. Contrary to "common sense" belief, satisfying marriages which encounter sexual problems they are unable to deal with can result in a break-up. Sex cannot save a marriage, but sex problems can destroy a marriage.

The limerance marriage (romantic love/passionate sex/idealization) is at high risk for divorce in the first five years due to sexual problems. They fail to make the transition from romantic love/passionate sex to a couple sexual style which involves strong, resilient desire. On the other extreme, alcoholic and spouse abuse marriages are very stable. When spouse abuse or drinking stops, the divorce rate goes up rather than down. The couple does not realize it will require time and effort to establish a satisfying, secure, and sexual marriage as a sober and non-violent couple. In addition, contrary to traditional assumptions, there are loving, satisfied, secure couples who experience sex dysfunction and low desire.

The healthiest marriage (long-term partnered relationship) is satisfying, secure, and sexual. Marriage meets needs for intimacy and security better than any other relationship (Johnson, 2008). Commit to put in time, energy, communication, and problem-solving to ensure each dimension remains positive in your life and relationship.

The role of sexuality is integral, but small—a 15–20% factor. Sexuality energizes your bond and reinforces feelings of desire and desirability. Whether married 2, 22, or 52 years you cannot take sexuality for granted. Sex cannot be treated with benign neglect. Desire/pleasure/eroticism/satisfaction needs attention in order to remain vital. Contrary to the traditional belief that sexual problems are a symptom of an individual or relationship problem, in most cases sex is part of an interactive, negative cycle. The sexual problem causes distress, robbing the relationship of intimacy and threatening relational security. Paradoxically, dysfunctional, conflictual, and especially avoidant sexuality has a more negative impact on the relationship than the positive role of healthy sexuality. A key to healthy sexuality is remaining an intimate sexual team through good and bad times. We examine each component in turn, remembering the whole is more than its component parts.

Satisfaction

Satisfaction does not mean dramatic feelings and a perfect relationship. Satisfaction involves acceptance of your own and your partner's strengths and vulnerabilities. This is the basis for a genuine respect, trust, and intimacy bond. Satisfaction includes respecting the spouse with his strengths and vulnerabilities, not just positive attributes. It involves acceptance of good experiences, fun times, pride in achievements, and the life you've built together. Respect also includes acceptance of the disappointments, defeats, hurts, poor decisions, and frustrations of your life and relationship. However, do not give problems control over you or your relationship.

Trust involves the belief that your partner has your best interest in mind. When there are problems, you trust he did not do something intentionally to hurt you. "He has your back." This doesn't mean you won't be disappointed, hurt, or frustrated, but his intention was not to hurt you. A respectful, trusting bond is the foundation for satisfaction.

Emotional intimacy nurtures your bond while sexual intimacy energizes it. Respect, trust, and commitment are the core components of a satisfying marriage. Emotional and sexual intimacy play an important role in making your bond special. Sexuality energizes and bonds your relationship. Relational and sexual satisfaction has an integral role in your relationship.

Security

Traditionally, couples assumed marital security—you stood by each other in good and bad times, "till death do us part." Marriage was about social acceptance, family, and stability. The quality of the relationship and the role of sexuality were downplayed. This led to mediocre and disappointing marriages which were stable, but unhealthy and unfulfilling, especially for women. Genuine marital security (which is more meaningful than stability) is based on a satisfying relationship. Women value secure relationships and families, not relationships which are neglectful, abusive, or destructive. That is why satisfying is the core dimension, and security is the second dimension. Life does not come with guarantees, but a genuine satisfying and secure marriage is of great value. The key to relational security is being present in good and bad times, trusting your partner's intentions, emphasizing a positive influence process, and a commitment to relational problem-solving. Realistically, 30% of marital problems are resolvable, 50–60% modifiable, and 10–20% need to be accepted, coped with, and worked around. A powerful myth leading to alienation and divorce is "if you love me, you'll change for me." Security involves accepting your partner and relationship with strengths and vulnerabilities. Security does not mean everything about your spouse and marriage is perfect. This is unrealistic and sets you up for alienation and divorce. Secure marriage is based on trust that you are committed, you continue to positively influence each other, being in the marriage brings out a healthy part of you, you love and respect your spouse, and you continue to grow individually and as a couple. Secure means not taking the relationship for granted or treating it with benign neglect. Your commitment is to a respectful, trusting, intimate marriage where you continue to influence each other and change individually and as a couple.

Sexual

Sexuality has a 15–20% positive role in your marriage whether you are 30, 40, 50, 60, 70, or 80. The function of sexuality is to energize your bond and reinforce feelings of desire and desirability. Sexuality is a shared pleasure, a means to reinforce intimacy, and a tension reducer to deal with life stresses as well as the stresses of a shared life. If you decide to have a planned, wanted child, sex with the goal of pregnancy is an aphrodisiac. Commit to confront the poisons of sex conflict, sex dysfunction, and especially sexual avoidance.

Couple sexuality is much more than intercourse. Sexuality involves sensual, playful, and erotic touch in addition to intercourse. A core concept to enhance sexual satisfaction is embracing the Good Enough Sex (GES) model of variable, flexible couple sexuality with a range of roles, meanings, and outcomes. Whether dysfunctional sex occurs once a month, once every ten times, or once a year, you turn toward each other in good and bad times. Do not fall into the traps of guilt, blame, and shame. Remain intimate and erotic allies.

Afterplay is an excellent strategy to enhance satisfaction. Couples ignore afterplay, and instead focus on intercourse and orgasm. You have just experienced an intense sexual encounter; enjoy an intimate, sensual, or playful afterplay experience which affirms your coupleness. Satisfaction is more than orgasm. Satisfaction involves reinforcing feelings about you as a sexual woman and being an intimate sexual team.

In the desire/pleasure/eroticism/satisfaction mantra, satisfaction is the second most important dimension. Sexual and relational satisfaction is not based on individual sex performance, but on sharing pleasure and eroticism as intimate allies. A key for satisfaction is accepting the range of roles, meanings, and feelings associated with couple sexuality. Especially important is to turn toward each other when you experience dissatisfying or dysfunctional sex.

Lori and David

Thirty-eight-year-old Lori just celebrated her tenth wedding anniversary with 37-year-old David. Their children are 7 and 5. They are committed to maintaining healthy couple sexuality throughout the parenting years. Lori and David take pride in "beating the odds" and integrating marriage, parenting, and sexuality.

Lori's parents had a stable marriage, but were not a satisfied or sexual couple. When Lori was 26 she had the courage to ask her mother personal questions. Lori was surprised and grateful that her mother answered honestly rather than give socially desirable responses. She was especially grateful for her mother's marital and sexual advice. Mother loved and respected Lori's father, but had been disappointed in their sexual relationship. She felt he was sexually selfish in the early years of the marriage, overemphasizing intercourse. Although they had been an affectionate couple, especially holding hands, her mother did not have her sexual voice—sex was the man's domain. Sadly, Lori's parents were in the one of three couples who stop being sexual after 60 because the man had lost confidence with erections and intercourse. Her mother misses intimacy and touching more than intercourse.

At first Mother had been hesitant toward David, but once Lori and David were a committed couple and Mother realized David was a kind man, she was supportive of the marriage and thrilled about becoming a grandmother. It was Mother who brought up present sexual issues with Lori. She urged Lori to value her marriage—intimacy, affection, pleasure, eroticism, intercourse, and afterplay. Lori wanted a satisfying, secure, and sexual marriage and her mother's prosexual stance was an important source of permission-giving. Mother urged Lori to be a first-class sexual woman. Further, she encouraged Lori to be a good model and sex educator for her daughter.

Lori and David had established an equitable and satisfying sexual relationship before their first child was born. After the limerance phase, they developed a Complementary couple sexual style. A key was valuing both mutual, synchronous sexual experiences and asynchronous sexuality. Asynchronous sex was usually better for David but was not at Lori's expense or the expense of their relationship. David treated Lori as his intimate and erotic friend. Lori's bridges to sexual desire were very different than David's. Accepting sexual preferences is an advantage of the Complementary sexual style. Lori enjoyed playful touch as a way to initiate sex while David preferred giving and receiving back-rubs as his bridge to desire.

Their Complementary couple sexual style was compatible with their Best Friend marital style. Lori valued their emotional relationship and secure marital bond. David valued that "Lori has my back" and was proud of their four-person family.

Maintaining vibrant, satisfying couple sexuality was a challenge not just because of young children, but dealing with the vicissitudes of their shared life. Lori had a stable job with a predictable income while David was an entrepreneur who had some great financial successes, but also very lean years. Lori's stable income gave them the ability to weather bad years, but caused anxiety for Lori. Over the ten years, David only out earned Lori three of those years although in total he earned much more. It was clear that David enjoyed his career more than Lori did hers. Healthy marriages are not perfect—all people and all marriages have their vulnerabilities.

Sexuality was a positive resource in dealing with the stresses and anxieties of life. Sex to share pleasure, reinforce intimacy, and energize your bond are prime functions. People underestimate the role of sexuality as a tension reducer.

With aging, feeling desire and desirable was especially important for Lori. Touch was her prime cue for desire—"responsive sexual desire." In addition, she maintained a positive (non-perfectionistic) body image. David had been quite athletic in his youth, although he no longer participated in competitive sports. A healthy couple activity was walking two—three miles a day. This was an enjoyable experience as well as time to share concerns and problem-solve. A healthy physical body contributes to sexual health. Although they drank, in the last few years they moderated alcohol consumption. Physically alcohol is a central nervous system depressant, although for many women and couples, alcohol has an inviting sexual role and reduces self-consciousness.

Last year David had his first experience with erectile anxiety. Lori's sexual response was variable and flexible, but David's had always been totally predictable. Lori did not want to overreact, but she didn't pretend the erection problem had not occurred. She wanted David to know that he didn't need to sexually perform for her. On a walk later that week, she told David that if sex didn't transition to intercourse she was enthusiastic about erotic experiences. He surprised her by saying let's try that this weekend. They created a mutual erotic scenario that was highly charged and fulfilling. David said he valued intercourse and being inside her, but sharing erotic sexuality was intimate and genuine. Lori affirmed that the best sex was mutual and synchronous. In addition, she valued encounters where she wasn't orgasmic—sometimes she would pleasure him to orgasm and other times intercourse was a "10" for him and a "6" for her. The bottom line for Lori was that they were genuinely engaged in sharing intimacy, pleasure, and eroticism. She didn't want David to panic or feel he had to apologize if sex did not transition to intercourse. He learned to accept sexual "blips" and enjoy a range of sexual experiences.

Lori had a friend who used sex as a form of manipulation. If her husband had an erection problem, she fellated him to orgasm. However, she manipulated him to buy her an extravagant pair of shoes as pay back. Lori wanted for her and David to be genuine sexual friends with no manipulation. Asynchronous sexual scenarios are healthy as long as it's not at the expense of the partner or relationship. Sexuality is not about emotional manipulation. Power struggles, manipulation, and hidden agendas subvert couple sexuality.

On their walks, Lori and David discussed problems and disagreements. They are aware of the guideline that 30% of problems are resolvable, 50–60% are modifiable, and accept that 10–20% are ongoing problems. An example of a resolved sexual problem was the decision for David to have a vasectomy. This made sex freer with the fear of an unwanted pregnancy eliminated. An example of a modifiable problem was that David enjoyed having an erotic story read aloud before a sexual encounter, but Lori did not find reading erotica sexually inviting. David assured her the erotic story was fantasy material, totally different than real-life couple sex. They agreed that when Lori was not interested in a mutually involving sexual experience, she would read an erotic story followed by intercourse where she was along for the ride. Lori did not feel a need for an asynchronous sexual encounter to "even the score." An example of a sexual problem which was not changeable was that David found being fellated to orgasm with Lori kneeling in front of him highly erotically charged. For Lori, this was a minus 3 on subjective arousal. She valued oral sex, both giving and receiving, but was turned off by that position and scenario. Rather than get stuck in a sexual power struggle—demanding, threatening, calling names—they accepted this difference with the assurance that David's disappointment and Lori's turn-off would not subvert their relationship. A key to satisfying sexuality is being intimate and erotic allies even when there are differences or the sex is dissatisfying or dysfunctional. Satisfying does not mean perfect. Accepting the spouse with personal, relational, and sexual vulnerabilities is a sign of a healthy relationship.

As she anticipates the future, Lori is confident they will be a sexual couple during the years of parenting adolescents and young adults. They want to enjoy each year of their children's lives, while looking forward to the "couple again" phase. They are committed to a satisfying, secure, and sexual marriage into their 60s, 70s, and 80s. Lori was more positive about aging than David, especially sex and aging. Their challenge was to maintain a genuine, human, interactive sexual relationship. David had a family history of heart problems and Lori had a family history of arthritis. They dealt with illness and problems caused by medication side-effects while remaining intimate and erotic. A crucial element of a healthy relationship is the belief "my partner has my back" practically, emotionally, physically, and sexually. There are no guarantees in life, but Lori and David's commitment to a satisfying, secure, and sexual marriage provides a solid foundation.

The Role of Sexuality

The essence of a marriage (or life partnership) is a respectful, trusting, emotional commitment. The role of sexuality is to energize your bond and reinforce feelings of desire and desirability. In addition, sex is a shared pleasure, enhances intimacy and attachment, and is a tension reducer to deal with the stresses of a shared life and the vicissitudes of life. If you decide to have a planned, wanted child, sex with the intention of pregnancy is an aphrodisiac. Sexuality has an integral role in a satisfying, secure relationship, but is not the dominant factor.

Be aware that sexuality has a multitude of roles, meanings, and outcomes. Often, the motivation and experience of the sexual encounter is different for your partner than for you. It can vary from experience to experience and change even within the same encounter. This is normal and healthy—you are not sexual clones of each other. Reinforce variable, flexible couple sexuality. The message of sex might be to heal an argument, reinforce feelings of desirability, reenergize you while dealing with the terminal illness of your sister-in-law, celebrate a career success, reinforce intimacy and attachment, cope with a boring time in life, a "port in the storm" after an argument with an adolescent, a way to celebrate a beautiful Fall day, share sadness after hearing of the death of a friend, or to acknowledge the specialness of your relationship.

Sometimes your partner has a very different agenda than yours. For one person sex is a positive way to end the day, for the other a tension reducer to induce sleep; he feels playful, for you a special moment before a difficult encounter with your mother-in-law; you act out angry feelings, he wants to feel reconnected; for you the frustration of not being pregnant, he feels valued as a lover; you show love, he experiences sex as a physical outlet. Understanding and accepting emotional and sexual differences (including those that do not follow traditional gender roles) affirms you as a sexual woman. Not all sex is or should be mutual, intimate, and serious. Playfulness, including asynchronous sexual encounters, is a sign of a healthy relationship.

Sexuality is a primary prevention strategy to ensure the "poisons" of dysfunction, conflict, and sexual avoidance do not destabilize your relationship. Paradoxically, the negative role of sexual problems is more impactful than the role of healthy sexuality. Sexual dysfunction, conflict, and especially avoidance drains intimacy and threatens relational viability. Maintaining desire/pleasure/eroticism/satisfaction is a wise emotional investment for a satisfying and secure marriage.

Exercise: Maintaining a Satisfying, Secure, and Sexual Marriage

Good intentions are important, but the most important factor is implementing sexual strategies and techniques. This exercise is done with your spouse (partner) in a personal, concrete, genuine manner—no manipulation or "politically correct" agendas. Remember, each dimension is important, but the whole is more than the component parts.

Be honest with your partner in discussing historical factors. What were your parents like as a marital and sexual model? Are there one or two couples (older or contemporaries) who provide a model of relationship vitality? What are your prime components for relationship satisfaction (loving feelings, a secure bond, children and family, a home, couple friends, career success, money, travel, sexuality)?

What is your experience in this relationship? When did you feel the most satisfied and what made you feel best? Be honest with yourself and your partner. What is your present level of satisfaction?

Your power to change is in the present and future. You can learn from the past but can't change the past. In terms of the present/future, list one (two at the most) problem that you believe is resolvable and would enhance satisfaction. List one (two at the most) problem you believe is modifiable and that would improve satisfaction. Lastly, what one (two at the most) problem do you need to accept and cope with while ensuring this does not control your view of the partner or relationship? A key for satisfaction is accepting your partner and relationship with vulnerabilities rather than demanding perfection.

What is your history regarding secure relationships? Did you grow up in an intact family? Do you have one—two models of secure marriage? Were those relationships satisfying? What is your expectation regarding your marriage (life partnership)? Do you value a secure bond? What would make your relationship secure? What can your spouse do to enhance marital security? The two dimensions most often cited are relational rituals and couple problem-solving. Rituals include anniversary celebrations, gifts, birthdays, and family traditions. These rituals are a public display that affirms your relationship is valued and honored. Problem-solving means addressing issues before a crisis. Prevention involves confronting issues, ideally before they become problems. Prevention is the most efficacious strategy. An example is if your career is advancing and you have become a "road warrior" (away from home three or more nights a week), talk about the challenges and how to cope. What can you do to affirm the new career reality, so your marriage and family remain satisfying and secure? If the changes are negative, what can you do so you have a valuable career with less stress and travel? Seldom is there a perfect resolution, but there are positive, realistic alternatives. These include taking advantage of the perks of your career travel such as planning a weekend as a couple before or after a business meeting.

With work, family, house, and community responsibilities, the dimension easiest to ignore is your sexual relationship. That is a very unwise choice. Sexuality cannot be treated with benign neglect whether you've been a couple for five, 25, or 45 years. You owe it to yourself and your relationship to maintain desire/pleasure/eroticism/satisfaction. Vibrant, satisfying couple sexuality is a healthy emotional investment. Every six months each partner initiates something new sexually. It could be purchasing a new lotion for a sensual body massage, playful sexual touching in front of a full-length mirror, a new position for oral sex, a different scenario mixing manual and oral stimulation to orgasm, switching intercourse positions three times during an encounter, using a different multiple stimulation scenario during intercourse, or a new afterplay scenario which reinforces emotional bonding. Each year you create two—four new sexual inputs. A key to satisfaction is valuing variable, flexible, unpredictable scenarios rather than expecting a perfect individual sex performance. Routine sex, even if functional,

> does not reinforce desire and satisfaction. Enjoy special sex and okay sex, synchronous and asynchronous sex, sensual scenarios and erotic scenarios, sex for tension reduction and loving sex, silly sex and intimate sex. Embrace couple sexuality with its multiple roles, meanings, and outcomes.

Summary

A satisfying, secure, and sexual relationship requires thought, energy, and communication. Embrace this as a positive, realistic goal. In past generations, the emphasis was on family and security. This resulted in stable but mediocre marriages. Women are concerned about the high divorce rate (although contrary to media hype the divorce rate peaked in the late 1970s and has decreased). The best way to ensure marital security is to focus on genuine satisfaction with yourself, your partner, and your marriage. Don't expect a perfect relationship, but you deserve a relationship worth having. This is especially true sexually. Couple sexuality has an integral 15–20% role of energizing your bond and reinforcing feelings of desire and desirability. The core of marriage is a respectful, trusting, emotional commitment. Sexuality is a crucial component in maintaining a vital, satisfying relationship. Sexuality is broad-based and variable including sensual, playful, and erotic touch in addition to intercourse. The desire/pleasure/eroticism/satisfaction mantra is important throughout life, including for aging couples. Quality female and couple sexuality enhances life satisfaction.

In a satisfying, secure, and sexual relationship the whole is more than the component parts. Sexuality has a vital 15–20% role in a satisfying, secure marriage. The core of marriage is a respectful, trusting, emotional commitment with female and couple sexuality energizing your bond. This book provides you with strategies and techniques to promote healthy sexuality for you and your relationship.

Appendix A
CHOOSING A SEX, COUPLE, OR INDIVIDUAL THERAPIST

This is a self-help book, not a do-it-yourself therapy book. Many women and couples are reluctant to consult a therapist, feeling that to do so is a sign of weakness, a confession of inadequacy, or an admission that their life and relationship are in dire straits. In reality, seeking professional help means that you realize there is a problem. You have made a commitment to address the issues and promote individual, couple, and sexual growth.

The mental health field can be confusing. Couple therapy and sex therapy are clinical subspecialties. They are offered by several professionals—psychologists, marital therapists, pastoral counselors, psychiatrists, social workers, and licensed professional counselors. The professional background of the clinician is less important than her competence in dealing with sexual, couple, and individual problems.

Many people have health insurance that provides coverage for mental health; thus, they can afford the services of a private practice therapist. Those who have neither the financial resources nor insurance could consider a university or medical school outpatient mental health clinical, a family services center, or a public mental health clinic. Most clinics have a sliding fee scale program.

When choosing a therapist, be direct in asking about credentials and arears of expertise. Ask the clinician what the focus of therapy will be, how long therapy is expected to last, and whether the emphasis is specifically on sexual problem or on individual, communication, or relationship issues. Be especially diligent in asking about university degrees and licensing. There are poorly qualified persons—and some outright quacks—in any field.

One of the best ways to obtain a referral is to call or look on-line for a professional organization such as a state psychological association, marriage and family therapy association, or mental health association. You can ask for a referral from a family physician, minister, imam, rabbi, or a trusted friend. If you live near a university or medical school, call to find what specialized psychological or sexual health services may be available.

For a sex therapy referral, contact the American Association of Sex Educators, Counselors, and Therapists (AASECT) at aasect.org. Another resource is the Society for Sex Therapy and Research (SSTAR) at sstarnet.org.

For a marital therapist, check the on-line site for the American Association for Marriage and Family Therapy (AAMFT) at therapistlocator.net.

If you are looking for a psychologist who can provide individual or couple therapy for anxiety, depression, behavioral health, and other issues we suggest the National Registry of Health Service Providers in Psychology at findapsychologist.org.

Feel free to speak with two or three therapists before deciding with whom to work. Be aware of your level of comfort and degree of rapport with the therapist as well as whether the therapist's assessment of the problem and approach to treatment make sense to you. Once you begin, give therapy a chance to be helpful. There are few miracle cures. Change requires commitment; it is a gradual and often difficult process. Although many people benefit from short-term therapy (less than ten sessions), most find the therapeutic process will require four months or longer. The role of the therapist is that of consultant rather than the decision-maker. Therapy requires effort on your part, both during the sessions and between sessions. Therapy helps you change attitudes, behaviors, and feelings. It takes courage to seek professional assistance. Therapy can be a tremendous help in assessing and ameliorating sexual, couple, and individual problems.

Appendix B

SUGGESTED READINGS

Suggested Readings on Female Sexuality

Brotto, L. (2018). Better sex through mindfulness. New York: Greystone.
Foley, S., Kope, S., & Sugrue, D. (2012). Sex matters for women (2nd ed.). New York: Guilford.
Heiman, J. & LoPiccolo, J. (1998). Becoming orgasmic. New York: Prentice-Hall.
Nagoski, E. (2015). Come as you are. New York: Simon and Schuster.

Suggested Readings on Couple Sexuality

McCarthy, B. & McCarthy, E. (2009). Discovering your couple sexuality. New York: Routledge.
McCarthy, B. & McCarthy, E. (2012) Sexual awareness (5th ed.). New York: Routledge.
McCarthy, B. & McCarthy, E. (2014). Rekindling desire (2nd ed.). New York: Routledge.
Metz, M. & McCarthy, B. (2010). Enduring desire. New York: Routledge.
Perel, E. (2006). Mating in captivity. New York: Harper Collins.
Snyder, S. (2018). Love worth making. New York: St. Martin's.

Suggested Readings on Male Sexuality

McCarthy, B. & Metz, M. (2008). Men's sexual health. New York: Routledge.
Metz, M. & McCarthy, B. (2003). Coping with premature ejaculation. Oakland, Ca.: New Harbinger.
Metz, M. & McCarthy, B. (2004). Coping with erectile dysfunction. Oakland, Ca.: New Harbinger.
Zilbergeld, B. (1999). The new male sexuality. New York: Bantam.

Other Significant Sexuality Readings

Maltz, W. (2012). The sexual healing journey (3rd ed.). New York: William Morrow.
Michael, R., Gagnon, J., Laumann, E., & Kolata, G. (1994). Sex in America. Boston: Little, Brown.
Snyder, D., Baucom, D., & Gordon, K. (2007). Getting past the affair. New York; Guilford.

Suggested Readings on Relationship Satisfaction

de Marneffee, D. (2018). The rough patch. New York: Scribner.
Doherty, W. (2013). Take back your marriage (2nd ed.). New York: Guilford.
Finkel, E (2017). The all-or-nothing marriage. New York: Dutton
Gottman, J. & Silver, N. (2015). The seven principles for making marriage work (2nd ed.). New York: Crown.
Johnson, S. (2008). Hold me tight. Boston: Little, Brown.
Love, P. & Stosny, S. (2008). How to improve your marriage without talking about it. New York: Three Rivers.
Markman, H., Stanley, S., & Blumberg, S. (2010). Fighting for your marriage (3rd ed.). San Francisco: Jossey-Bass.
McCarthy, B. & McCarthy, E. (2004). Getting it right the first time. New York: Routledge
McCarthy, B. & McCarthy, E. (2006). Getting it right this time. New York: Routledge.

REFERENCES

Allen, E., Atkins, D., Baucom, D., Snyder, D., Gordon, K., & Glass, S. (2005). Intrapersonal, interpersonal, and contextual factors in engaging in and response to extramarital involvement. Clinical Psychology: Science and Practice, 12, 101–130.

Basson, R. (2001). Using a different model for female sexual response to address women's problematic low sexual desire. Journal of Sex and Marital Therapy, 27, 395–403.

Baucom, D., Pentel, K., Gordon, K., & Snyder, D. (2017). An integrative approach to treating infidelity in couples. In J. Fitzgerald (Ed.) Foundations for couple therapy (pp. 206–215). New York: Routledge.

Brotto, L. & Luria, M. (2014). Sexual interest/arousal disorder in women. In Y. Binik & K. Hall (Eds.) Principles and practice of sex therapy (5th ed., pp. 17–41). New York: Guilford.

Brotto, L. & Woo, J. (2010). Cognitive-behavioral and mindfulness-based therapy for low sexual desire. In S. Leiblum (Ed.) Treating sexual desire disorders (pp. 149–164). New York: Guilford.

Feldman, H., Goldstein, I., Hatzichriston, D., & McKinley, J. (1994). Impotence and its medical and psychological correlates. Journal of Urology, 151, 54–61.

Fine, C. (2017). Testosterone rex: Myths of sex, science, and society. New York: Norton.

Foley, S., Kope, S., & Sugrue, D. (2012). Sex matters for women (2nd ed.). New York: Guilford.

Frank, E., Anderson, A., & Rubinstein, D. (1978). Frequency of sexual dysfunction in "normal" couples. New England Journal of Medicine, 299, 111–115.

Gillespie, B. (2017). Sexual synchronicity and communication among partnered older adults. Journal of Sex and Marital Therapy, 43, 441–455.

Graham, C. (2014). Orgasm disorders in women. In Y. Binik & K. Hall (Eds.) Principles and practice of sex therapy (5th ed., pp. 89–111). New York: Guilford.

Hamann, S., Hermann, R., Nolan, L., & Wallen, K. (2004). Men and women differ in amygdala response to visual stimuli. Nature Neuroscience, 7, 411–416.

Heiman, J. (2007). Orgasmic disorders in women. In S. Leiblum (Ed.) Principles and practice of sex therapy (4th ed., pp. 84–123). New York: Guilford.

Heiman, J. & Lo Piccolo, J. (1988). Becoming orgasmic. New York: Prentice-Hall.

REFERENCES

Heiman, J., Long, J., Smith, S., Fisher, W., Sand, M., & Rosen, R., (2011). Sexual satisfaction and relationship happiness in midlife and older couples in five countries. Archives of Sexual Behavior, 40, 741–753.

Hillman, S. (2008). Sexual issues and aging within the context of work with aging patients. Professional Psychology: Research and Practice, 39, 290–297.

Hyde, J. (2005). The gender similarities hypothesis. American Psychologist, 60, 581–592.

Johnson, S. (2008). Hold me tight. Boston: Little, Brown.

Kleinplatz, P. & Menard, A. (2007). Building blocks toward optimal sexuality. The Family Journal, 15, 72–78.

Laumann, E., Paik, A., & Rosen, R. (1999). Sexual dysfunction in the United States. Journal of the American Medical Association, 262, 537–544.

Leiblum, S. (2002). After sildenafil: Bridging the gap between pharmacological treatment and satisfying sexual relationships. Journal of Clinical Psychiatry, 63, 17–22.

Lindau, S., Schumm, L., Laumann, E., Levenson, W., O'Muircheartaign, C., & Waite, L. (2007). A study of sexuality and health among older adults in the United States. New England Journal of Medicine, 357, 762–774.

Masters, W. & Johnson, V. (1970). Human sexual inadequacy. Boston: Little, Brown.

McCarthy, B. (2015). Sex made simple. Eau Claire, WI.: PESI Publications.

McCarthy, B. & Bodnar, L. (2005). The equity model of sexuality. Sexual and Relationship Therapy, 20, 225–235.

McCarthy, B., Koman, C., & Cohn, D. (2018). A psychosocial model for assessment, treatment, and relapse prevention for female sexual interest/arousal disorder. Sexual and Relationship Therapy, 33, 353–363.

McCarthy, B. & McCarthy, E. (2009). Discovering your couple sexual style. New York: Routledge.

McCarthy, B. & McCarthy, E. (2014). Rekindling desire (2nd ed.). New York: Routledge.

McCarthy, B. & Metz, M. (2008). Men's sexual health. New York: Routledge.

McCarthy, B. & Pierpaoli, C. (2015). Sexual challenges with aging. Journal of Sex and Marital Therapy, 41, 72–82.

McCarthy, B. & Ross, L. (2017). Integrating sexual concepts and interventions into couple therapy. In J. Fitzgerald (Ed.) Foundations for couples' therapy (pp. 355–364). New York: Routledge.

McCarthy, B. & Wald, L. (2013). New strategies in assessing, treating, and relapse prevention of extramarital affairs. Journal of Sex and Marital Therapy, 39, 493–509.

McCarthy, B. & Wald, L. (2016) Finding her voice. Sexual and Relationship Therapy, 31, 138–47.

Meana, M. (2010). Elucidating women's (hetero)sexual desire. Journal of Sex Research, 47, 107–122.

Metz, M. & Epstein, N. (2002). Assessing the role of relationship conflict in sexual dysfunction. Journal of Sex and Marital Therapy, 28, 139–164.

Metz, M., Epstein, N., & McCarthy, B. (2017). Cognitive-behavioral therapy for sexual dysfunction. New York: Routledge.

REFERENCES

Metz, M. & McCarthy, B. (2004). <u>Coping with erectile dysfunction</u>. Oakland, CA.: New Harbinger.

Metz, M. & McCarthy, B. (2010). <u>Enduring desire</u>. New York: Routledge.

Metz, M. & McCarthy, B. (2012). The Good Enough Sex (GES) model. In P. Kleinplatz (Ed.) <u>New directions in sex therapy</u> (2nd ed., pp. 212–230). New York: Routledge.

Mosher, D. (1980). Three psychological dimensions of depth of involvement in human sexual response. <u>Journal of Sex Research</u>, 16, 1–42.

Muise, A. & Impett, E. (2015). Good, giving, and game. <u>Social Psychological and Personality Science</u>, 6, 164–172.

Nagoski, E. (2015). <u>Come as you are</u>. New York: Simon and Schuster.

Nelson, T. (2012). <u>Getting the sex you want</u>. New York: Quiver.

Nobre, P. (2017). Treating men's erectile problems. In Z. Peterson (Ed.) <u>The Wiley handbook of sex therapy</u>, pp. 40–56. New York: Wiley/Blackwell.

Perel, E. (2006). <u>Mating in captivity</u>. New York: Harper Collins.

Reid, R. & Jorgensen, R. (2017). Cybersex and pornography. In J. Fitzgerald (Ed.) <u>Foundations for couples' therapy</u> (pp. 93–102). New York: Routledge.

Rosen, R., Miner, M., & Wincze, J. (2014). Erectile dysfunction: Integrating medical and psychological approaches. In Y. Binik & K. Hall (Eds.) <u>Principles and practice of sex therapy</u> (5th ed., pp. 61–85). New York: Guilford.

Sims, K. & Meana, M. (2010). Why did passion wain? A qualitive study of married women's attributions for declines in sexual desire. <u>Journal of Sex and Marital Therapy</u>, 36, 360–381.

Ter Kuile, M., Both, S., & van Lankveld, J. (2012). Sexual dysfunction in women. In P. Sturmey & M. Herson (Eds.) <u>Handbook of evidence-based practice in clinical psychology: Vol. II. Adult disorders</u> (pp. 413–436). Hoboken, NJ.: Wiley.

Weiner, L. & Avery-Clark, C. (2017). <u>Sensate focus in sex therapy: The illustrated manual</u>. New York: Routledge.

Weeks, G. & Gambecia, N. (2000). <u>Erectile dysfunction: Integrating couple therapy, sex therapy, and medical treatment</u>. New York: Norton.

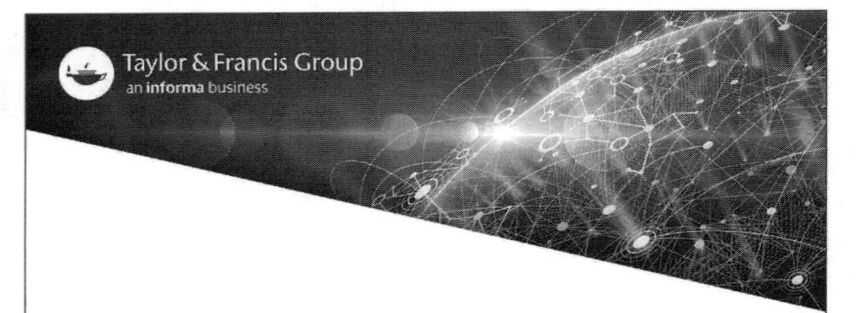

Taylor & Francis eBooks

www.taylorfrancis.com

A single destination for eBooks from Taylor & Francis with increased functionality and an improved user experience to meet the needs of our customers.

90,000+ eBooks of award-winning academic content in Humanities, Social Science, Science, Technology, Engineering, and Medical written by a global network of editors and authors.

TAYLOR & FRANCIS EBOOKS OFFERS:

- A streamlined experience for our library customers
- A single point of discovery for all of our eBook content
- Improved search and discovery of content at both book and chapter level

REQUEST A FREE TRIAL
support@taylorfrancis.com

Routledge
Taylor & Francis Group

CRC Press
Taylor & Francis Group